CARING FOR YOUR
TODDLER

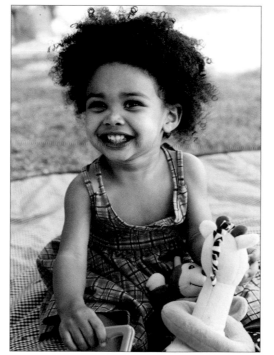

Raising your child the way nature intended

Kim Davies

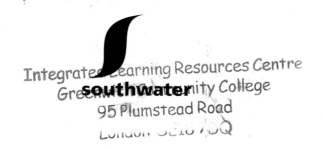

southwater

This edition is published by Southwater, an imprint of Anness Publishing Ltd, Hermes House, 88–89 Blackfriars Road, London SE1 8HA; tel. 020 7401 2077; fax 020 7633 9499

www.southwaterbooks.com; www.annesspublishing.com

If you like the images in this book and would like to investigate using them for publishing, promotions or advertising, please visit our website www.practicalpictures.com for more information.

UK agent: The Manning Partnership Ltd; tel. 01225 478444; fax 01225 478440; sales@manning-partnership.co.uk
UK distributor: Grantham Book Services Ltd; tel. 01476 541080; fax 01476 541061; orders@gbs.tbs-ltd.co.uk
North American agent/distributor: National Book Network; tel. 301 459 3366; fax 301 429 5746; www.nbnbooks.com
Australian agent/distributor: Pan Macmillan Australia; tel. 1300 135 113; fax 1300 135 103; customer.service@macmillan.com.au
New Zealand agent/distributor: David Bateman Ltd; tel. (09) 415 7664; fax (09) 415 8892

Publisher: Joanna Lorenz
Editorial Director: Helen Sudell
Executive Editor: Joanne Rippin
Designer: Nigel Partridge, Cover Design: Adelle Morris
Photographer: Scott Morrison

With special thanks from the author to Eliza and Jake for the practical experience, and to Jonathan Bastable for the fatherly perspective. Thanks, also to these parents for their honesty and wisdom: Melanie Davies, Hilary Silverwood, Marta Scott, Juliet Cox and Sally Harper.

Photographs in the book were taken by Scott Morrison, and are the property of Anness Publishing Ltd. Photographs also taken by: Jo Harrison: 26b, 29b and John Freeman: 58-59 all.

Thank you to the parents and children who took part in the photoshoots: Elizabeth and Oliver Allen, Evie Beswick, Heather, Imogen and James Call, Irena and Rose Andrews, Jancien and Arabella Lambeth, Jenny and Lucy Rose, Freddie Lorenz, Kirsty and Olivia Innes, Marion Demoissier and Louisa Swann, Rose and James Wallis, Sam Beattie and Sienna Brown.
Thanks to the following agencies for supplying additional images: Alamy: 8b,13b, 15tl, 16b, 17br, 18, 19tl, 25b, 27b, 30, 31 both, 41tr, 47tr, 52b, 57tr &b, 61tr, 81tl, 84tl, 88b. Corbis: pp51t, 64, 65 both.

ETHICAL TRADING POLICY
Because of our ongoing ecological investment programme, you, as our customer, can have the pleasure and reassurance of knowing that a tree is being cultivated on your behalf to naturally replace the materials used to make the book you are holding. For further information about this scheme, go to www.annesspublishing.com/trees.

Previously published as part of a larger volume, *Baby & Childcare the Pure and Natural Way*

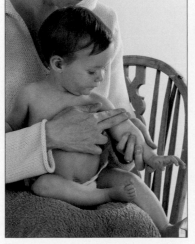
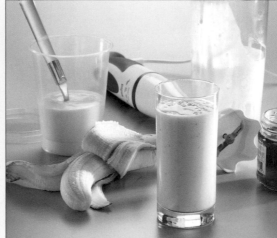
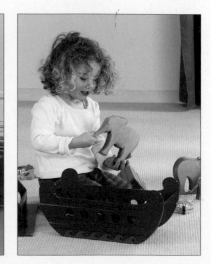

Contents

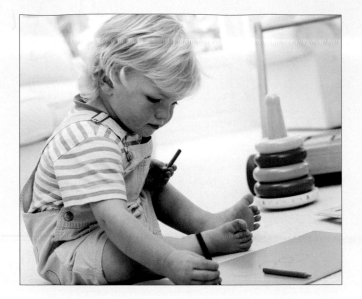

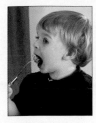
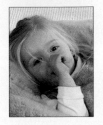
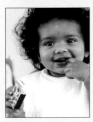
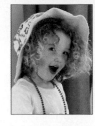
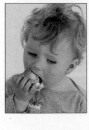
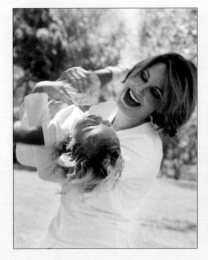

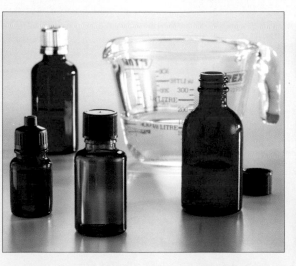

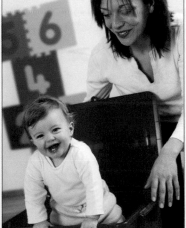

Introduction

Toddlers are amazing creatures: they are curious, strong-willed, unselfconscious, as changeable as the weather, and always ready to share love and laughter. The time that a baby grows into a toddler is a time of huge change, and often both the child and the parent can feel overwhelmed by the rapid changes that are taking place. For the parent there is the sudden realization that their control is not absolute, and they have to adapt their care and nurturing to include a level of compromise and negotiation. For the child, the desire to be more independent and to do things for him or herself now becomes much more important. The preschool years are also important foundation blocks for the rest of a child's life. Physical development depends on the healthy diet, sleep and exercise that you offer your toddler, social development will be enhanced by a daily routine that involves interaction with other children and adults, and their mental development will be stimulated by how much you talk to and play with them.

This book is intended to help you adapt to this period in your child's upbringing, to deal with the new challenges

One of the most important developments for your pre-school child is potty training. It is important that this is a natural process, not one that is forced or pressurized.

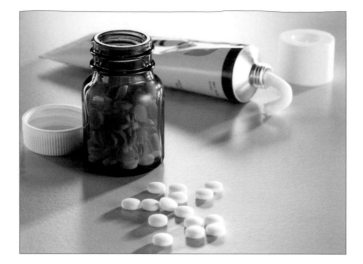

Homeopathic treatments, such as arnica tablets and cream, are a drug-free way to treat minor ailments.

and enjoy to the full the fun and energy your toddler will exude. The central theme of the book is how to make choices that are soundly natural, responsibly ecological and roundly sensible. Childcare, like any other social activity, is subject to fashion – but this book is not a trendy guide to green parenthood, and has no ideological axe of its own to grind. The aim of the book is primarily to help you to bring up your child in a way that does as little

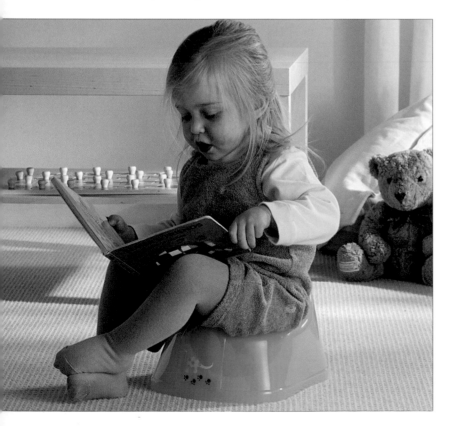

You don't need to spend huge amounts of money on toys; dressing up in your old clothes will give a child hours of fun.

Natural remedies can help you treat some of the common ailments that all children often experience.

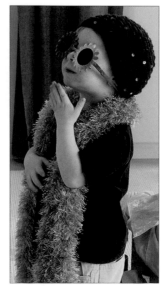

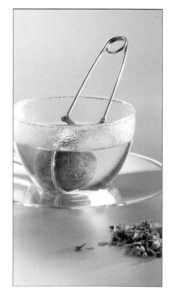

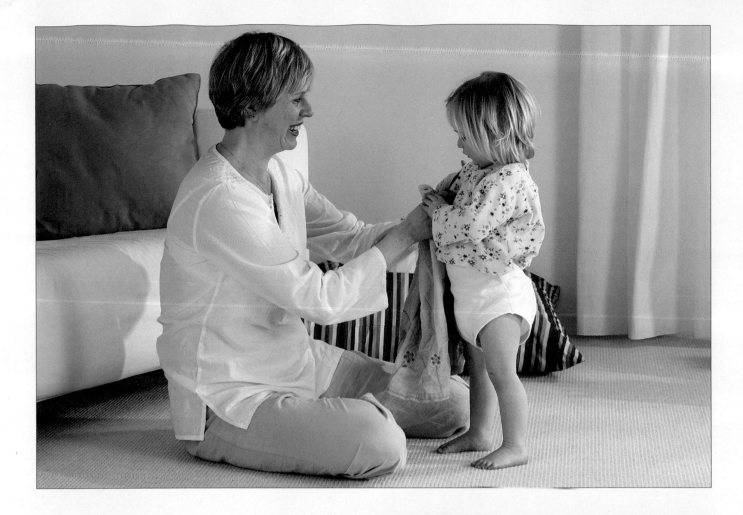

how to introduce the potty and encourage your child to use it. Another common life change that may happen in your first child's toddler years, one over which they have absolutely no control, is the arrival of a younger brother or sister. This is something that has to be carefully managed, but with a little tact and forethought the growth of your family can be as joyful a time for your older child as it is for you.

Always remember that your toddler's growing independence is a positive thing, even if it might make life trying from time to time. It is delightful to watch your little child wash his or her own face with a flannel or to put their wellingtons on the wrong feet, and it gives him or her great pleasure too. So as far as possible, try to nurture your child's natural enjoyment in doing things for themselves.

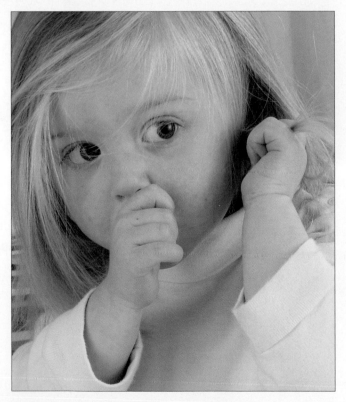

Top: It's fun to see your child gradually working out how to do things for him or herself. Most children want to help get themselves dressed from an early age.

However independent toddlers may seem at times, they are still babies emotionally. Your child may become more needy if a new baby arrives on the scene.

Washing and keeping clean

As your toddler gets older, you begin the process of teaching him or her to become more independent, starting to feed, wash and take care of themselves, or at least becoming aware of what is involved. Your toddler may embrace these new activities with enthusiasm – little children take great delight in doing things for themselves, especially if they perceive a task as a grown-up one. They are also inveterate copiers, and will enjoy performing tasks and jobs with you rather than only under instruction.

CLEAN HANDS

Toddlers inevitably get grubby, and an evening bath is the easiest way to get them clean after a busy day in the sandpit and the garden. In between times, though, it is important that young children wash their hands before meals and after using the potty or helping to take off a used nappy (diaper), so it is a good idea to instil regular handwashing habits early on. Your child will still need your help until about the age of three.

Get a step so that your toddler can reach the washbasin, and teach him or her the difference between the hot and cold taps. Demonstrate how to turn on the cold tap. Teach your child not to touch the hot one – and consider reducing the temperature of your hot-water supply to less than 55°C/130°F to prevent accidental scalding. Begin by lathering your own hands and then gently rub the soap bubbles all over your toddler's. Make it fun by blowing the bubbles into the air, or by having hand-washing races.

A toddler may positively enjoy washing his or her hands just like mummy and daddy. Choose a natural soap without harsh chemicals.

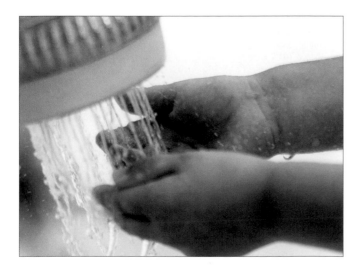

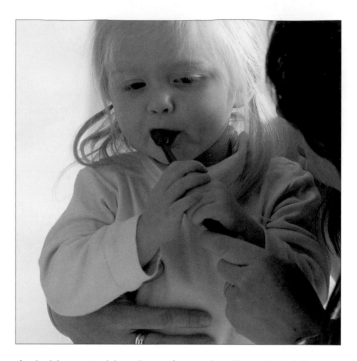

As babies get older, they often enjoy the twice-daily ritual of cleaning their teeth. But they can't brush them properly on their own until they are much older.

GETTING CLEAN

Your toddler's skin is very delicate so it is important to avoid harsh soaps or bath products. A handful of oats gathered in a piece of muslin makes a good alternative to soap, and you can avoid using shampoo altogether if you wish and simply rinse your child's hair with water: the natural oils in the hair will keep it clean. If you want to use products, choose natural ones free from chemicals, and limit hair washing to once or twice a week.

Many toddlers dislike having their hair washed. If you have this problem, you can sponge the hair to get rid of clumps of food. But from time to time, you will have to wash it. If you use shampoo, choose a gentle one that won't sting if it gets in your child's eyes.

NAIL CARE

It's easier to keep fingernails and toenails clean if they are short – long nails can harbour dirt and germs. But most toddlers hate having their nails cut and it is almost impossible to do this safely if your child keeps wrenching his or her hand or foot away. The best solution is to cut the nails when your child is asleep, but you could also try doing it as part of a game such as "This little piggy". Child-sized nail clippers are usually the best way to cut small nails, but some children prefer to have them filed.

TOOTHBRUSHING

If your toddler is reluctant to let you clean his or her teeth, try letting him or her do yours first or brush a favourite toy's "teeth". Tooth cleaning is important, so persevere even if it is difficult. Try doing it after supper rather than just before bedtime if it becomes a flashpoint. Take your toddler with you when you visit the dentist. Children don't need a check-up until they are about two, but it is good to make the dentist's surgery and the "special chair" a familiar environment long before that.

BATH TIME

You don't have to hold your toddler in the bath like a baby, but you do still need to be vigilant. Remember that small children can drown in just a few centimetres of water and in a few moments, so don't ever leave a toddler in the bath unattended or in the care of an older child, however sensible he or she may seem. Encourage your toddler to remain seated in the bath – to prevent slipping – and teach him or her to avoid touching the hot tap (wrap a wet flannel around it as an additional safety precaution).

FEAR OF THE BATH

Most children love baths, but some toddlers become frightened of the water or develop a dislike of the sound and sight of water disappearing down the plug hole. It is as if they fear they will go down with it. Treat these fears seriously – forcing a reluctant child to get in the bath will do more harm than good, and it's not a problem to give your toddler sponge baths for a few weeks. After a while, though, you will want to encourage your child back into the bath. Be sure to go slowly.

Start by getting in the bath together (if possible, have someone else on hand to lift the child in and out). Invest in a few new and exciting bath toys – wind-up toys are particularly good for this – to encourage play in the water. Once your toddler is feeling more relaxed about getting into the bath with you, try putting him or her in alone. But let the child stand up if this is easier (with you holding on as he or she could easily slip). Try scooping water over the child's ankles, then legs, bottom, tummy and back while he or she continues to stand.

Have plenty of toys in the bathwater: empty, cleaned shampoo or bubble-bath bottles, natural sponges, a flannel and plastic pots and beakers are good. Let your toddler bend down to pick a toy up. When you think he or she is ready, put the child in a sitting or kneeling position and then quickly provide a distraction by setting off a moving toy or pouring water from one pot into another. Keep the bath short, let your child hold on to you and have lots of physical contact during the bath, and cuddles afterwards. Don't pull the plug out until your child is out of the water (or out of the room if necessary) if it makes him or her feel scared.

MILK BATH

Here is a fragrant mixture to add to a toddler's bath. Milk is gentle on the skin, and an ideal medium for diluting essential oils. Mix the bath milk just before you need it because it won't keep.

100ml/3½fl oz full-fat milk
3 drops lavender essential oil
3 drops neroli essential oil
5ml/1 tsp blue or red food colouring (optional)

Pour the milk into a bowl or jug and add the essential oils, then the food colouring if you are using it. Stir to mix and pour the mixture into a warm bath.

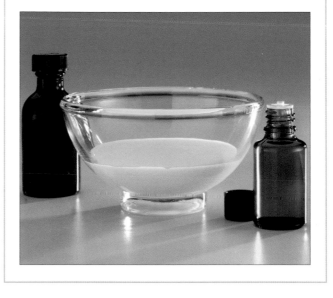

Children usually love baths, and if your child shows some reluctance it is more than likely to be a short-lived phase. He or she will soon be enjoying them again.

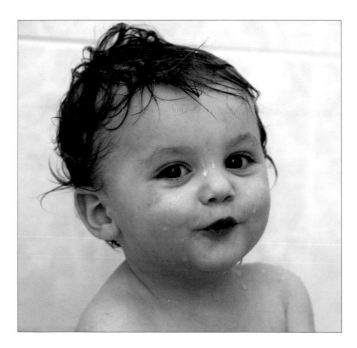

A healthy diet for toddlers

Toddlers have busy lives and small stomachs, so they need to eat little and often. Three meals a day – breakfast, lunch and dinner – is a convenient routine to aim for, but you will also need to offer a mid-morning and mid-afternoon snack to keep your child going between meals. Don't expect your toddler to eat the same amount every day – his or her appetite will vary hugely. It's completely normal for a young child to refuse food on some days and to eat extra helpings on others.

A VARIED DIET

You probably won't be able to get your child to eat perfectly balanced meals every day, but if you offer a wide variety of healthy food, this should add up to a reasonably good mixed diet over a week or so. It is very normal for children to refuse all but a few chosen items from time to time, but so long as your toddler is eating one or more foods from each group, you don't need to worry. Ideally your child will eat a good mixed diet consisting of the following foods each day.

Five or more servings of fruits and vegetables. Try to include as many types as possible.

Four or five helpings of starchy foods such as rice, potatoes, pasta, couscous or quinoa. Don't be tempted to put a young child on a high-fibre diet: wholegrains are bulky and they fill young children up without providing the necessary nutrients.

One or two servings of protein foods such as lean meat, fish, pulses, eggs or nuts. If your child doesn't eat meat or fish, give two servings of other protein a day.

Milk 500ml/17fl oz up to the age of two years; 350ml/ 12fl oz after two, or the equivalent in cheese, fromage frais, yoghurt and so on. Use plain, full-fat dairy products: fruit yoghurts often contain lots of sugar and small children shouldn't eat low-fat dairy products.

Some iron-rich foods the best sources are red meat, chicken or fish, but tofu, beans and lentils, leafy green vegetables, dried fruit, fortified breakfast cereals and bread also contain some iron. Eating vitamin C-rich foods such as brightly coloured fruits and vegetables at the same time helps the body to absorb the iron.

Some healthy fat – olive oil and avocados are good sources. Give oily fish at least once a week.

DRINKS

Drinking lots of water with snacks and at mealtimes will help to keep your toddler's digestion healthy. Juice isn't really necessary, but if you want to give it to increase your child's vitamin intake, make sure that it is well diluted (one part juice to ten parts water for young toddlers, slightly stronger for older ones). Fizzy and sweetened fruit drinks and even fruit juice will coat the teeth in sugary liquid, so, ideally limit drinks to milk and water.

> **FOODS TO AVOID**
> Don't add sugar or salt to your young child's food.
> Avoid the following altogether:
> • Raw eggs
> • Whole or chopped nuts (grind or flake them)
> • Shark, swordfish or marlin
> • Unpasteurized milk or cheese.

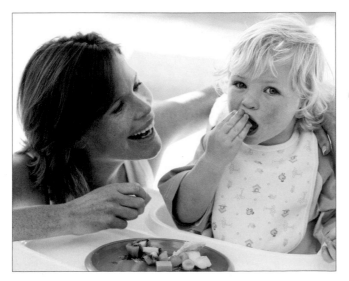

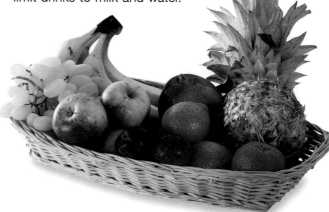

Left and above: It's important to encourage healthy eating habits from an early age. Fortunately most children love fruit – try to give them as wide a variety as possible and keep trying new types.

SWEETS AND CRISPS

It is much easier to ensure that your child eats healthily if you limit the intake of empty calories. All children love crisps and sweets, but they have no nutritional value, and they tend to ruin a child's appetite for more wholesome foods. That is not to say that such foods should be banned altogether (although it is a good idea to hold off introducing them for as long as you can), only that you and your child should see them as occasional treats. Set an example yourself by eating healthy foods: if you enjoy chocolate and biscuits after lunch, then your child will want some too.

If you do give sweets, choose kinds that dissolve quickly in the mouth rather than sticking to the teeth – chocolate instead of chewy sweets, for example. And get your child to eat them in one go: a lot of sweets eaten in a few minutes will actually do less harm to the teeth than eating a few at staggered intervals through the day. If possible, get your child to drink a glass of water afterwards, or to eat a piece of cheese, which helps to neutralize the effect of sugar on teeth.

DAIRY PRODUCTS

Milk is a good source of calcium (which is needed to build strong bones and teeth), vitamin A (for healthy skin, eyes and immune system) and fat (needed for energy), as well as protein. If you have stopped breastfeeding, you can now give full-fat cow's or goat's milk as your baby's main drink, or you can stick to follow-on formula milk if you prefer. Choose organic milk and dairy products whenever possible. Don't give skimmed milk or low-fat dairy products to children under five, because they need plenty of calories. You can start giving semi-skimmed milk to children over two, so long as they are eating and growing well. If your toddler stops drinking milk, give three servings of cheese, yoghurt, fromage frais or milk-based dishes a day. Here are some suggestions.

- Porridge or pancakes made with full-fat milk.
- Homemade fruit milkshakes or yoghurt smoothies.
- Dhal or soup with yoghurt stirred in.
- Quick "rice pudding" made with cooked rice and plain yoghurt (it doesn't need sugar).
- Mini sandwiches made with Cheddar or cream cheese as a mid-morning snack.
- Cooked vegetables with cheese sauce.
- Mashed potatoes made with lots of milk and butter.
- Chunks of Cheddar, hard goat's cheese or Edam, served with slices of fruit.
- Greek or plain yoghurt.

NON-DAIRY ALTERNATIVES

There is a lot of debate about the health benefits of eating dairy foods, and it is clear that some children (such as those with milk-allergy-related eczema) are better off

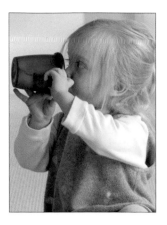

Leave a cup of water close by when your child plays so he or she can help him or herself.

avoiding them altogether. If you want to restrict the amount of dairy products you give your child because of intolerance or for other reasons, here are some good alternative sources of calcium. A paediatric dietician can advise you about planning your child's diet to ensure that it is not deficient.

- Unsweetened rice milk or soya milk with added calcium (don't give sweetened soya milk, which is bad for the teeth). But be aware that some children who are intolerant of dairy products are also intolerant of soya.
- Tofu (made with soya beans) or beans.
- Ground nuts and seeds.
- Canned salmon and sardines (with bones), mashed well.
- Leafy green vegetables: spinach, kale, greens.
- Dried apricots and figs.

Offer your child only healthy food choices for as long as you can. This is much easier if you eat healthily too – your child is much more likely to eat a piece of fruit if he or she sees you eating one.

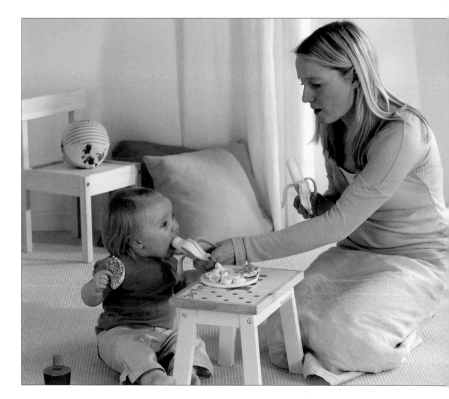

Helping your toddler to enjoy food

Toddlers are often picky eaters and a child's eating habits can cause parents a great deal of stress. But there are many ways you can help to give your child a positive attitude to food. As a general rule, it is best to let your toddler's appetite be your guide. You will naturally find yourself gently coaxing your child to eat vegetables, but it is pointless to try to force a child to eat more than he or she wants. If your toddler is a healthy weight and has plenty of energy, then he or she is almost certainly getting enough. Check with a health professional if you are not sure.

HAPPY EATING

After the age of one your child can eat pretty much everything you eat (with the exception of very salty or spicy foods) provided it is chopped small enough to manage easily. This means you can include your toddler in family mealtimes and make eating a sociable activity. Push the highchair up to the table, and later get a booster seat so that he or she can sit comfortably at the table.

It's best if your child sits down for snacks and there is less chance of choking that way. He or she will love food to be served on a toddler-size table or low stool.

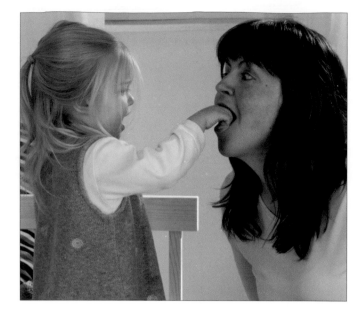

Children like to copy their parents and to try what you eat. Eating together and sharing food is a good way to make food an enjoyable part of life.

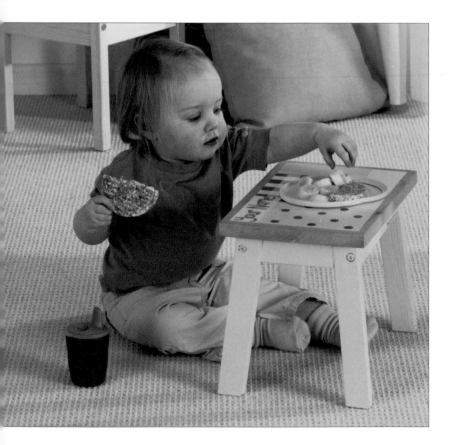

If you like to eat a little later than a young child's blood-sugar levels will allow, treat your meal as an extra snacktime for him or her. Don't wait until your child is so tired or hungry that he or she is cranky before eating. Having regular meals and snacktimes will help to regulate his or her energy levels.

Let your child have a spoon and feed himself or herself as soon as he or she seems willing. Having control over how much and what is eaten helps to foster a positive attitude towards food. You can get forks with rounded tines for older toddlers. Your toddler will be more willing to eat an amount that looks manageable than a huge pile of food, so serve small portions. You can always give your child a second helping if he or she wants one.

LIKES AND DISLIKES

Be tolerant about food fads. Most children go through stages when they reject foods they have previously enjoyed, or when they have certain rules about how food must be presented. It is common, for example, for children to dislike "mixed-up" food and to insist that each element of a meal be served in a separate pile that doesn't touch the others. It's often good to humour these fads, but talk to a health professional if you think your child's attitude to food is extreme.

Young children like to copy grown-ups (or older children) and studies show that children whose parents eat lots of fruits and vegetables tend to eat them too. So chop a raw pepper at snacktime and share it with your toddler, or offer some green vegetables off your plate. But children should never be forced to eat foods they dislike or to finish a meal if they are no longer hungry. Remember your own childhood meals. If you were made to eat a food you disliked, or told to sit at the table until you had scraped the plate clean, you may recall how it didn't make you eat any better. Worse still, the child will realize that refusing to eat is a good way of getting your attention and may use this as a way of exercising independence.

Don't assume that your child doesn't like a new food if it's initially rejected. Children may need to be offered a food ten times or more before it becomes familiar enough for them to eat it. So keep serving that portion of red pepper or spinach alongside other foods that your child will eat. It's very tempting to get out, say, bread and cheese if your toddler rejects the meal you have prepared. This doesn't do any harm from time to time, but if you do it often you may be storing up problems for the future.

If your toddler picks at meals, consider whether he or she is having too much milk or snacks at other times. Limit milk to the recommended daily amount, and don't give a snack within an hour of a meal – if a toddler is really hungry, it is better to bring the mealtime forward.

FRUIT AND VEGETABLES

Here are some ways to get your toddler eating plenty of fruits and vegetables.

• Serve fruit at all or most mealtimes. For example, chopped banana or pear in morning porridge; slices of apple after lunch; and peaches and yoghurt after supper.

Make mealtimes calm, happy times. Avoid discussing difficult issues or commenting on your child's eating habits in a negative way.

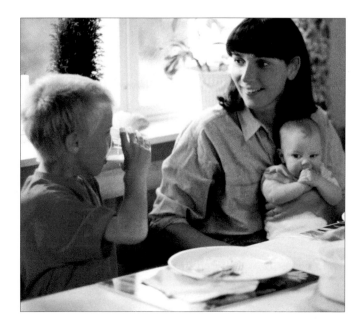

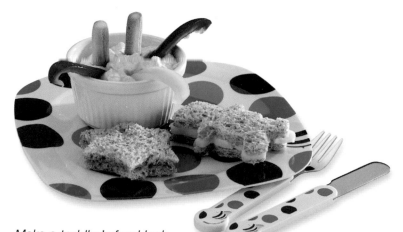

Make a toddler's food look appetizing. Offer brightly coloured vegetables with every meal – red and yellow peppers alongside breadsticks with a dip, say. Sometimes you may like to use biscuit cutters to make little sandwiches in the shape of teddy bears or stars.

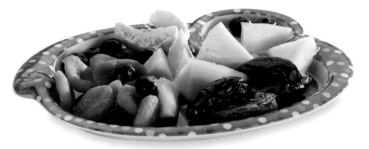

Serving fruit at every snack time will help to up your child's vitamin intake. Encourage them to try exotic fruits as well as the standard apples and bananas.

• Make sure you always have two or three different kinds of fresh fruit in the house. Keep homemade fruit purées in the freezer and serve them alone or stirred into yoghurt or plain fromage frais.
• Give your child raw vegetable sticks as snacks or to keep him or her amused while waiting for a meal – sticks of carrot and cucumber are good served with a dip: hummus or guacamole are good healthy options.
• Include vegetables in every savoury meal. Ideally have one green vegetable and one other vegetable to get a good range of vitamins.
• Keep vegetables in the freezer so you don't run out. If you can't find ready-frozen organic vegetables, make your own: chopped and lightly steamed carrots, green beans, baby sweetcorn and broccoli all freeze well.
• Stir chopped, puréed or grated vegetables into rice, mashed potato, dhal or tomato sauce for pasta. Grated carrot or courgette (zucchini) go well in pancakes.
• Remember that children don't have preconceptions about which foods should be served together. It is fine to use vegetable soup as a pasta sauce or to stir chopped dried fruit into a lamb casserole. And if you are resorting to a tin of (low-salt, low-sugar) baked beans, stir in some peas or spinach to increase the vitamin content.

Preparing for toilet training

Learning to use a potty is an important part of growing up. Teaching your child to do it can be an easy process – provided that you wait until he or she is ready. If you start too early, it will take longer and there will be more accidents along the way. Most children are potty trained somewhere between the ages of two and a half and three years, but some take longer or are ready earlier. Most children master control over the bowel before the bladder, and will be dry during the day long before they can stay dry all night long. Remember, however long the journey, they all get there in the end.

IS MY CHILD READY?

Children start to become aware that they are doing a wee or poo at around 18 months. At this stage, they may clutch themselves and look down at a puddle of wee if they are naked – a sign that they understand they have produced it. It usually takes another year or more before they know in advance that they need to go to the toilet and have the necessary control to wait for a few minutes. When this happens, your child is ready to start potty training, provided there are no other major changes going on – for example, you are about to move house, a new baby is expected or your child is starting nursery. Here are the signs to look out for.

- Your child tells you that he or she is about to do a wee or poo – whether it is communicated in words, by facial expression or by actions.
- Your child remains dry after a nap or for more than two hours at a time.
- Your child makes it clear he or she objects to having a dirty or wet nappy (diaper).
- Your child is able to understand simple instructions, and knows what toilet-based words such as "wee" and "poo" (or whatever words you decide to use) mean.
- Your child is happy to try sitting on the potty and understands what it is for. Some children may ask to use the potty if they see their friends doing it.
- Your child has mastered all the physical skills needed to use a potty successfully – that is, walking well, sitting down and standing up unaided, and pulling his or her underwear on and off.

WHAT YOU NEED FOR TOILET TRAINING

A potty. Choose a sturdy one that won't tip over when your child sits on it and is easy to clean. If your child already knows about potties, he or she might like to choose one – narrow the choice down to two or three different types. **Proper cotton pants.** Choose pants that your toddler will enjoy wearing, perhaps with a favourite character or motif on. You'll need at least ten pairs to begin with.

Training pants. Some parents find towelling training pants useful because they retain wee or poo, but can still be pulled up and down like proper pants. You can use them as a halfway stage, or as a safeguard when out and about. That way, your child will feel wet after an accident – which can help with potty training – but you won't have to deal with a public puddle. Change them quickly and emphasize how nice it is to be clean and dry. It is better not to use disposable trainer pants as they wick away the wetness too efficiently. This results in your child getting the treat of wearing pull-down pants without having to stay dry for the privilege.

Steps and a child seat for the toilet. Some children don't like the idea of a potty, but are keen to use the big toilet. If this is the case, you will need to buy a set of child's steps, so that your child can get on to the toilet on his or her own. A child's toilet seat is vital, so that the toddler feels secure when sitting on the toilet.

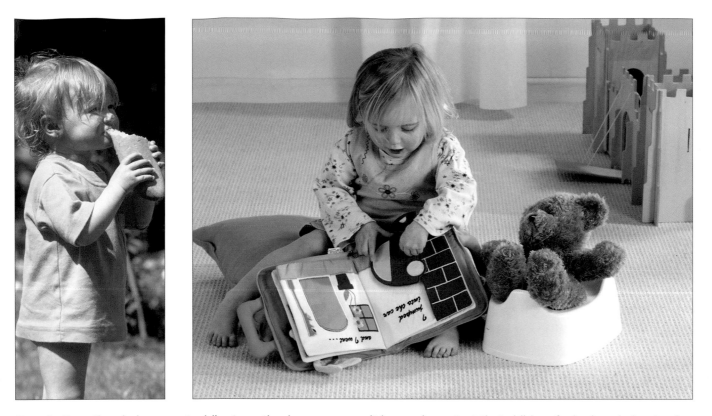

Bare-bottom time helps your toddler to notice how weeing feels. Your child may view the puddle with great interest months before he or she is ready for the potty.

It is very important that children feel relaxed about using the potty. Keep it in the living room before beginning to use it and watch how your child includes it in play.

PREPARING YOUR CHILD

It is important that your toddler feels good about going to the toilet. He or she probably gives some telltale signs that mean a poo or wee is coming: going red in the face, squeezing the legs together, standing on tiptoes, clutching the crotch and so on. Tell your child what is happening in a calm but interested way, and don't look disgusted when you are changing a nasty nappy.

If you feel able to, it is a good idea to let your child see you use the toilet – take the opportunity to explain what you are doing. If you have older children, ask them if your toddler can watch them go to the toilet, too, but don't put them under pressure – they have a right to privacy if they want it. It's particularly helpful if a girl sees mummy use the toilet, and a boy sees what daddy does.

GETTING READY

The first step is to get your child used to having a potty around. Keep it in the bathroom near the toilet, but bring it out to the play area from time to time too.

• Get a colourful book about a child learning to use the potty, so that your child starts to understand what it is for.

• Play at putting teddy or dolly on the potty. Later on, your child may like to have teddy sitting on the travel potty while he or she sits on the real one.

• Put a few toys or books around the potty to encourage the child to sit on it while fully clothed. Don't press or, worse still, force your child to sit on it. It is vital that he or

she feels comfortable at every stage of potty training and that you are relaxed about it.

• Once your child is happily sitting on the potty, put it back in the bathroom and keep it there. He or she may like to sit on it while you use the toilet. You can also try casually suggesting that your child sits on it when naked before a bath – but don't push this.

As your child gets accustomed to the potty as part of their play, you can start to encourage them to sit on it themselves as part of the game.

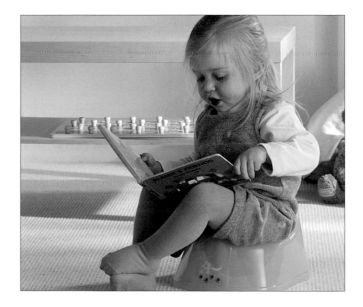

Toilet training problems and special circumstances

The process of toilet training can sometimes create a lot of tension. Parents may feel bad if their child is the last in a group to be toilet trained, or they may be under pressure from family members who insist that their children were trained before the age of two. It is important to know that some children (particularly boys) are not ready for potty training until they are over three. If in doubt, it is better to wait than to force the pace.

If you feel anxious about toilet training, it is worth seeking reassurance and advice on how to proceed. Remember that lots of children have problems with potty training, and an experienced health professional will almost certainly have already encountered any problem that your child has.

SETBACKS

Even children who have been successfully potty trained can start having accidents again, or suddenly refuse to use the potty. This can sometimes be due to a physical problem, such as a urinary infection, so see a doctor to check if this is the case.

If your child is in daycare, take several changes of pants and clothes when you are potty training. Discuss your method with nursery staff to avoid giving conflicting messages or using different terminology.

More often, setbacks are the result of emotional upset, such as the child being unsettled by an event such as a house move. Deal with the mess as calmly as you can and consider whether you need to offer some extra help for a while. Your child may want you to stay with him or her while using the potty, or something may be needed to refocus the child's attention – new pants, for example, or some stickers for the potty, and probably lots of extra loving attention too. If the problem persists for longer than a week or two, you may want to consider going back to nappies for a while and starting potty training afresh in a few weeks. Seek advice from your health visitor.

Children sometimes have a sudden increase in accidents simply because the activity they are involved with is more interesting than going to use the potty. If you think this is what is behind an apparent step backwards, say that it is not right to wait; your child must use the potty when he or she needs to go. Revert to asking often whether the child needs a wee, and put him or her on the potty at regular intervals for a while. But don't get angry.

SOILING

Some children may hold back from doing a bowel movement because they are frightened of doing it in the potty. Eventually they will soil themselves, because they can't hold on forever, and this adds to their distress. Be

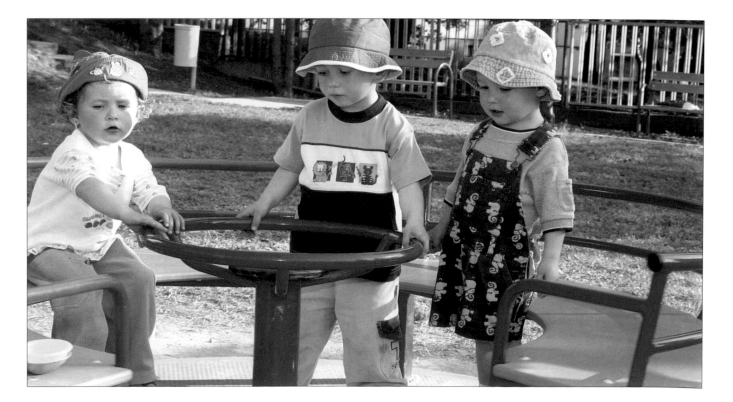

TRAINING TWINS

If you have twins, you may find it easier to train one before the other, or to train them simultaneously. Both methods can work well, so long as the children are ready for potty training when you start, are treated as individuals and their progress is not compared. You will need two potties, and it may be a good idea to get them in different colours and to let each twin personalize their own. However, some twins will want potties that are exactly the same.

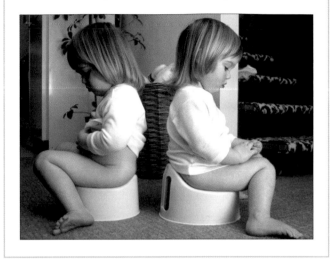

calmly sympathetic as you clean the child up and explain briefly that this happened because he or she held on. This may be enough to prevent it happening again. Children are more likely to do it if they are unsettled, so give extra attention and cuddles. Again, it can help if you stay with a child who is using the potty, and if you let the child leave the room to play before you flush the faeces away.

Sometimes soiling is the result of constipation, as liquid stools may leak past the hard ones. The child may not even realize that a bowel movement is happening until it is too late. If your child soils regularly and you think constipation may be the cause, seek professional help. Your child may need a laxative, but this should only be given under medical advice. Once the initial problem has been sorted, you'll also need to take steps to prevent your child from becoming constipated again.

CONSTIPATION

If your child is reluctant to do a bowel movement in the potty and is passing hard pellets, adding more fibre to the diet can help. Increase the amount of vegetables and fruits, and get the child eating some prunes and dried fruits. It is also helpful to increase the amount of wholegrain cereals and bread. Avoid bananas for a while and give the child plenty of water to drink. Excess intake of milk can sometimes be a factor in constipation, so keep an eye on how much your child drinks. See a health professional if the problem persists.

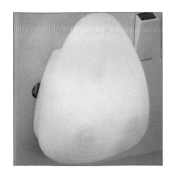

Using a plug-in light in the hallway may encourage your child to use the toilet in the night. It gives a very gentle glow and can provide reassurance as well as enough light to guide the child to the toilet.

BEDWETTING

Many young children wet the bed occasionally. Most grow out of this by the age of five, but if your child is wetting the bed often, you may want to try the following.

- Consider if you have started night-time training too early – talk to a health professional if you are not sure.
- If your child has been dry but has now started wetting the bed, he or she may be upset about something. It's also possible that a urinary infection or threadworms are to blame, so see a doctor if the cause is unclear.
- Try not to be cross. Remember that your child is not doing this on purpose, and the more calmly you deal with the problem the easier it will be to solve. Shaming or telling off a child will only make things worse. Don't accidentally encourage your child either by, say, bringing him or her into your bed whenever it happens.
- Restrict drinks after 5.00pm – but make sure the child has enough fluid earlier in the day.
- Put a cover on the mattress to minimize the damage, and have fresh sheets and pyjamas on hand so you can clean everything up quickly.
- Wake your child up for a wee when you go to bed. Most children will go back to sleep quite easily.
- Make sure the way to the bathroom is well lit during the night or have a potty in the child's room if he or she is afraid to go to the bathroom in the night.

If your child won't do a bowel movement in the potty, but is happy to wee in it, try some extra inducement. Fill a special "potty box" with small gifts – crayons, stickers, balloons and little toys – and let the child pick one every time he or she manages to do a poo in the potty.

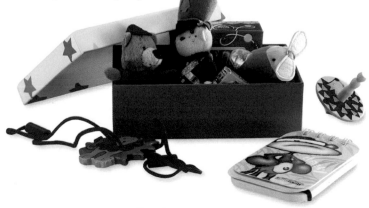

Crying, behaviour and sleeping

❝ A good bedtime and sleep routine is one of the key factors that will help your child to behave reasonably. ❞

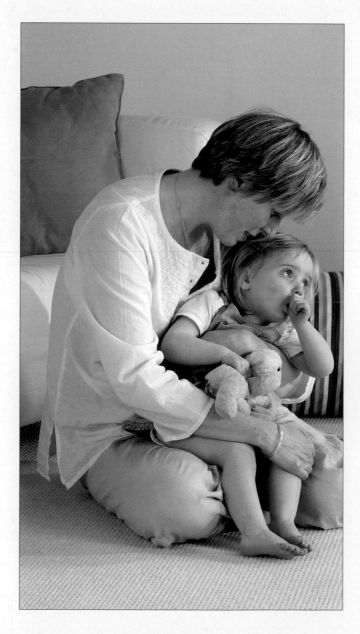

The years between the ages of one and three are probably the most emotionally tumultuous in a child's life. This is a time when your toddler may zig-zag between tearful neediness and fierce insistence on doing things his or her own way. Your child wants to be independent, but lacks the physical skills to manage without help. He or she wants to have you near all the time, but is furious if you try to show the way. This contrariness is what makes hard work of the job of parenting a toddler, but it is also what makes it such an absorbing experience. There are few things more fulfilling than sharing in your child's glee in attainments that bring him or her ever closer to the world of bigger children and adults: walking to the shop, repeating "Woof" whenever a dog appears, wielding a fork or successfully negotiating the stairs.

Your toddler will be testing all kinds of boundaries, so this is the time to start laying down some basic rules. There are simple ways to help your child to behave well when wilfulness spills over into conflict

Tantrums can abate as suddenly and rapidly as they arise, leaving that furious struggling child sobbing, frightened and in need of a loving cuddle.

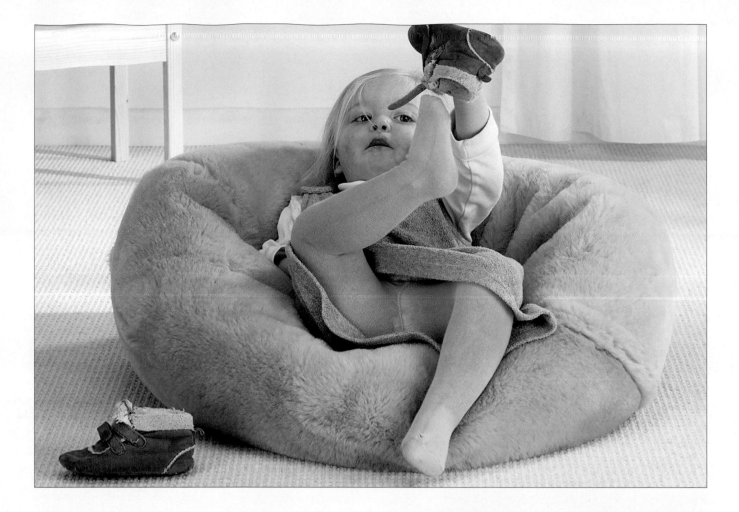

or tantrums. Some children have personalities that are more intense than others, and a very determined, creative or sensitive child is more likely to have tantrums than one who is naturally laid-back or timid. But the way you respond to crying may also play a part in determining how tantrum-prone your child becomes. A good bedtime and sleep routine is one of the key factors that will help your child to behave reasonably. A regular sleep pattern is the foundation of a daily schedule: get this right, and your toddler is more likely to be happy and equable during the day.

In this chapter there are ideas and techniques to help your child manage his or her moods and sleep well at night. Not all the suggestions will work for every child – it is up to you to choose the ones that suit you and your family.

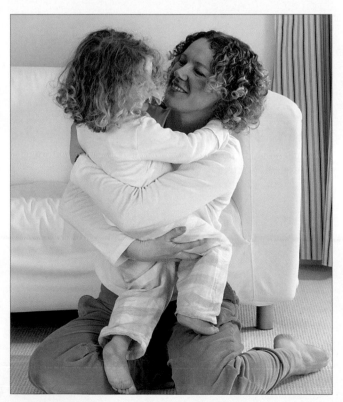

Top: That drive towards independence is ever-present, but toddlers don't understand the easiest way to go about things and need lots of tactful help.

Although parenting a toddler can be hard work, it is fantastically rewarding too. Nothing beats the affection you get from your child.

Why toddlers cry

Toddlers may cry several times a day, and their upset may seem out of all proportion to the cause. But it is important to remember that your toddler simply isn't equipped to deal with difficulties yet. Young children don't have the experience to know that what they are feeling is rage, still less that it will soon pass. Crying is the only way they have of coping with unpleasant emotions. It is also still a key mode of communication, since they can't express their needs or feelings accurately with their limited vocabulary.

FRUSTRATION

There is a huge gap between the things your toddler wants to do and what he or she can manage. Frustration can be positive because it helps to spur a child on to new developmental achievements. But it isn't a comfortable feeling and it can quickly lead to tears of rage. Your toddler will also feel frustrated when prevented from doing something that is enjoyable – a small child doesn't understand, after all, why drawing on walls is bad or why he or she should have to get out of the bath.

FEAR, ANXIETY AND LACK OF ATTENTION

The world can seem a strange and overwhelming place to a young child. Toddlers often develop a fear of, say, the bath, dogs, the dark or certain noises, and will cry when they encounter them. Separation anxiety is normal in toddlers, who want to stay close to their carers and resist being left with other people. Your toddler may no longer cry when you leave a room, but may become distraught if you go out or leave him or her at nursery.

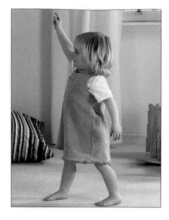

It's important to give growing children lots of ways to release physical energy, it can help to reduce tantrums too. You don't have to go outside for this, try putting on some lively music and having a dance around the house. It will probably improve your mood too.

Most children will cry when they are told off, because they fear the withdrawal of love from you. To an extent, this is a necessary part of socialization, but it is important to reassure children that you still love them even when they are naughty. Young children have an insatiable need for attention. If you are absorbed in another task, chatting on the phone or – worst of all – cuddling a friend's baby, your child may start to cry or behave badly simply because he or she wants you to play.

HOW YOU CAN HELP

Some crying is inevitable, and part of your child's way of expressing themselves, but you can minimize mood swings, and perhaps avoid a tantrum, as follows.
Rest. Your toddler will cry much more readily when tired. Make sure he or she is getting enough sleep and do all you can to help your child relax: a walk in the buggy or some quiet play on your lap can be almost as good as a sleep in restoring a toddler's spirits.

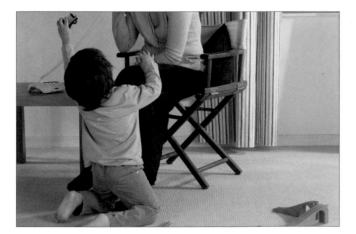

However happily absorbed in a game, your toddler is bound to want your attention the minute he or she notices that you are otherwise occupied.

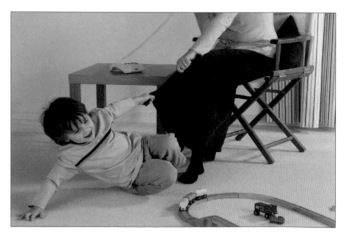

Not getting his or her own way can lead to an increasing sense of frustration and may easily end in an explosive tantrum.

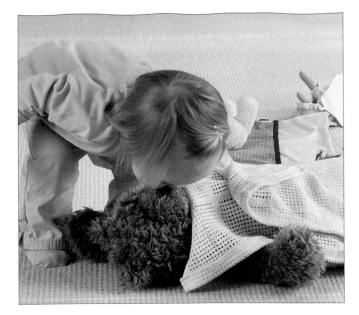

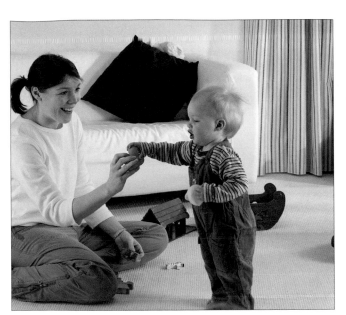

Toddlers have no sense of time and no conception of anyone else's needs. So don't expect them to stop playing just because you need to move on. Give a child time to adjust by saying you will be leaving in a while.

Fuel. Low blood-sugar levels or dehydration make children (and adults) irritable and fretful. So give regular meals and snacks, with plenty of water to drink. Avoid sugary snacks, which give an initial boost but soon lead to a dip in energy and mood.

Physical release. Toddlers have lots of energy that they need to expend. Go on at least one outing a day, more if your child is very active or has regular tantrums. Toddler gym classes are great, but simple outings or indoor activities such as dancing can work just as well.

Sympathy. Be swift to reassure your child if he or she has a bump or is frustrated when playing with a toy. Be sympathetic about any fears – don't dismiss them as "silly" or, worse, try to force your child to confront the thing that is frightening. Your child will almost certainly get over any fear more quickly if you are reassuring.

Independence. Toddlers are determined to do things for themselves, but don't always have the skills necessary to carry it out. Lend a hand where possible, but be tactful – your child will resent being "babied". Offering a few simple choices – does he or she want an apple or a banana, say, or to wear trousers or shorts, can help a child feel that he or she has some small mastery of the daily routine, and will boost self-confidence.

Preparation. Don't demand a sudden change of activity. If your child is involved in a game but it's time to leave, give five minutes' warning, and then a one-minute warning, too, so he or she is prepared for the change.

Distraction. If your toddler starts to get upset, try starting a new game or activity, exclaiming at something you see out of the window, singing a song and pulling faces, or taking the child out for a change of scene.

One of the most charming things about toddlers is their desire to be helpful. Your child may wipe the highchair tray or pass you something when you ask for it. This is a good behaviour trait to encourage.

DELIBERATE CRYING

Toddlers gradually become aware of what crying can achieve and its effect on adults, and realize they can use it to get something that they want – think of young children whining for sweets in the supermarket. At first, this is not so much devious as experimental: your child is naturally going to test all the methods available to see what works and once he or she discovers crying can get results, a toddler is bound to try it on from time to time. It is up to you to differentiate between genuine upset and deliberate whining, so you don't reward bad behaviour.

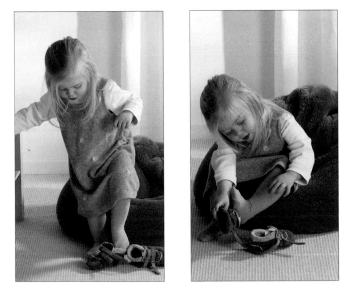

Help your toddler to do as much as possible for himself or herself, even though it is bound to take longer. If a child wants to try putting on his or her own clothes, leave plenty of time to get ready.

Dealing with tantrums

All children have to learn what is and what isn't acceptable behaviour, and this learning process starts early. Toddlers are driven by their own desires and have little sense of other people's feelings, so you can't expect them to know how to behave by themselves. Your child needs clear guidance from you.

Be reasonable. Have as few rules as possible, but put your foot down when it is important.

Be consistent. Make sure you, your partner and any other carers stick to the same basic rules.

Set a good example. If you shout at your child or your partner, your child is likely to copy you.

Encourage your child to ask nicely rather than to whinge or shout for what he or she wants.

REINFORCING GOOD BEHAVIOUR

Acknowledge pleasant behaviour with praise and extra attention and ignore bad behaviour when you can. It is easy to get into the habit of telling a child off for being naughty but ignoring all the good things. If your child gets most attention from you for being "naughty", then that is what he or she will be. So stop your child from doing naughty or dangerous things, but don't tell him or her off unless it is really necessary.

Avoid confrontation when you can. If your child doesn't want to walk up the hill, say, suggest you have a walking race. If he or she wants to play with a sibling's favourite

Older children may throw a fake tantrum. This is usually because they have discovered tantrums are a successful tactic.

If your child has lots of tantrums, try keeping a diary to help you pinpoint what the triggers are and then try to avoid them.

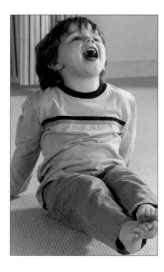
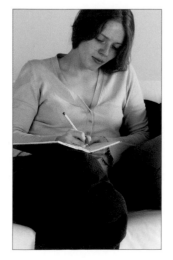

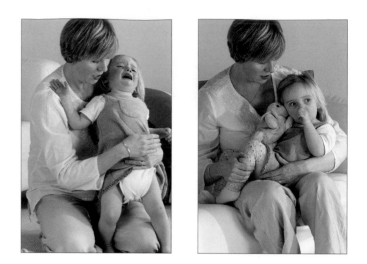

Young children may do best being held during a tantrum; they are then in the best place for a kindly cuddle and calming words once the temper abates.

toy, take it away but give the toddler something as a substitute. If you do need to tell a child off, get down to the child's level and make eye contact. Use a firm, low voice (don't shout) and tell the child the behaviour was unacceptable. Say: "Hitting people is wrong. We do not hit people." Don't say "You are naughty."

TEMPER TANTRUMS

Almost all young children will have temper tantrums from time to time and some intense toddlers have several a day. Tantrums often start at around 18 months, coinciding with a surge in independence. They may continue until

TACTICS FOR DEALING WITH A TANTRUM

When a tantrum starts, do the following.
- Make the environment safe so your child cannot get hurt or hurt other people.
- Some toddlers are helped by being held firmly, but this can make others even angrier.
- Do not engage: do not talk or argue with your child. Either stay nearby but avoid eye contact (read a book) or remove yourself altogether, if it is safe to do so. Deprived of an audience, your child may call a halt to the tantrum more quickly.
- If you are out, pick your child up and go somewhere quieter – your car, a quiet part of the park, a different room in grandma's house.
- Never, under any circumstances, give in.

the age of three or older, when children develop the language skills they need to express themselves. Adults have their own strategies for dealing with anger and fear, some healthy, some not. But all that young children feel is the overwhelming physical sensations that these emotions bring with them – tense body, tingling in the fingers and a head that feels it is about to explode.

A tantrum is usually the result of frustration, or sometimes of fear. It is more likely to happen if a child is also feeling overwhelmed, fatigued, hungry or thirsty. You may be able to prevent tantrums by avoiding key triggers or by diverting your child's attention once you see them building up, but once a tantrum has started there is usually nothing that you can do to stop it: a child in the midst of an explosion of rage is out of control, beyond reason, punishment or reward.

Waiting until the storm blows over is difficult, even for the most laid-back of parents. Most tantrums are awful to watch: children may fling themselves around the room, throw themselves down and drum their heels on the floor, hit out at you and scream. Some children yell so hard and for so long that they make themselves vomit, and others hold their breath until they turn blue in the face or even faint. Rest assured that it is impossible for children to stop themselves breathing for long; the body's natural reflexes step in well before any harm is done.

COPING WITH A TANTRUM
Remember that however hard it is to witness your child in the throes of a tantrum, the experience is worse for the child, who may be genuinely terrified by the maelstrom of emotion that has welled up inside, and who will need your comfort and reassurance as soon as it is over. Calm is the best weapon you have. If you get angry, or show amusement, you will simply add fuel to the fire. And if you

A temper tantrum can erupt in a moment, and is sometimes the only way young children know to release the pent-up rage inside them.

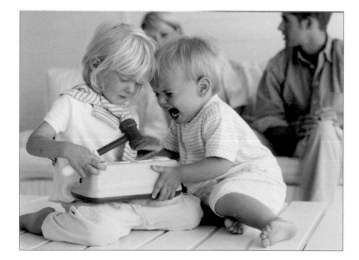

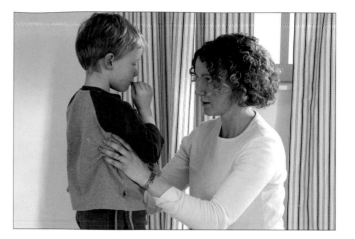

The underlying cause of tantrums is often the child's inarticulacy. As the child grows older, he or she will be able to talk more easily about his or her frustration.

try to draw a screaming toddler into a discussion, you are wasting your time. Your basic aim is to show your child that the tantrums do not frighten you (as they frighten the child), they do not push you into doing what your child wants and they do not stop you loving him or her.

Above all, do not give in. If the tantrum was precipitated by your refusing your child a treat, say, do not suddenly offer it, even if you now think your refusal was unwarranted. If your child learns that tantrums are a good way of getting what he or she wants, there are bound to be more of them. For the same reason, don't "reward" a toddler for a tantrum by producing a treat afterwards.

Don't punish your child, either. When the tantrum stops, be ready to have a cuddle if he or she will allow it, and say that you are glad the tantrum has stopped. Reassure your child that you love him or her but you don't like that behaviour. Then continue with your day as planned; don't cancel arrangements because your child has been naughty.

With an older child, consider talking about the behaviour afterwards. Your child may benefit from discussing the anger, how the tantrum felt and ways he or she could alert you to the onset of this feeling next time. You will help your child to become emotionally literate if you put a name to the uncomfortable sensations of frustration or anger he or she has experienced.

Think about triggers for tantrums and consider ways to avoid them. For example, if the tantrums occur in the supermarket, make sure your child is well rested and has had a snack and a drink before you go shopping. Keep the child occupied: for example, pass him or her the groceries to put in the trolley. And keep the trip as short as possible. If your child has lots of tantrums, give him or her oily fish at least once a week. It may also be worth trying a fish-oil supplement specially formulated for children: a large UK study found that taking fish oils reduced tantrums and difficult behaviour.

Toddlers and sleep

Most young children need 10–12 hours sleep a night, but this won't necessarily be in one long stretch. If your child isn't sleeping through the night, take heart from the fact that you are not alone: around one in three toddlers has difficulty settling at bedtime or wakes frequently through the night.

DAYTIME NAPS

Most toddlers continue with day-time naps until they are at least two and a half. A one year old will probably still need two naps a day: one in the morning and one in the early afternoon. Over the next few months, he or she will probably drop one of these and the second will probably go a year or so later.

Making these transitions can be difficult. Two naps may leave your one year old wide awake at bedtime, but one may leave a child overtired and cranky by the end of the day. When your child drops the last nap, you may want to try having an early supper and then putting him or her to bed at, say, 6.00 instead of 7.00 pm. Be patient at this time, it won't last long. Arrange a quiet interlude at the time when the nap used to be. Your toddler may be happy to lie on the bed for a while, or sit down for a story.

HOW MUCH SLEEP?
Children vary in how much sleep they need, but this is how long an average toddler will sleep over a 24-hour period:
At one year – 13.5 hours
At two years – 13 hours
At three years – 12 hours

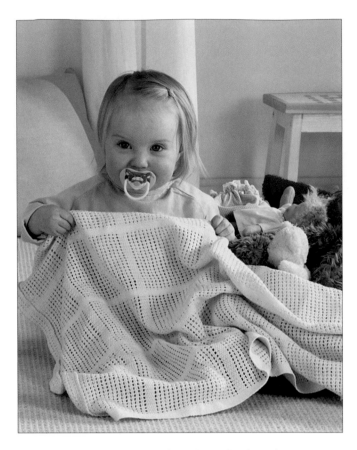

Children become attached to dummies but they can interfere with speech development. Using them at nap times only will make it easier to get rid of them later on.

MOVING INTO A BIG BED

A toddler can move from a cot to a proper bed any time between the ages of 18 months and three and a half years. There is no rush – it's better to wait until your child is keen to try a big bed rather than to push him or her into it too soon. If your child has learned to climb out of the cot, but isn't ready for a bed, make sure the mattress is on the lowest level and check that he or she is not using toys as steps. Put a duvet on the floor to provide a soft landing and move any furniture away. Consider keeping the side down so the child can climb out safely. But if your child can easily climb out of the cot, or is too big to sleep comfortably in it, it is probably time to make the move. It is also a good idea to move your child into a bed before you start night-time potty training, since he or she may need to get up in the night.

Most toddlers will carry on needing a sleep during the day, to ensure that in 24 hours they are getting around 12 hours sleep in total.

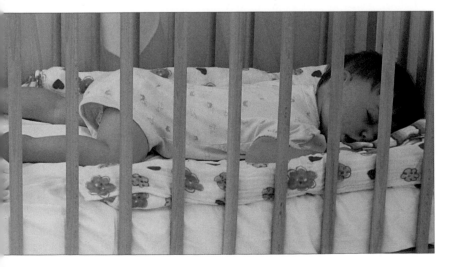

Here are some ways to help your child make the move from the cot happily.

- Don't do it when your child is undergoing any other big change, such as getting used to a new carer.
- If a new baby is due, either make the move to a bed two or three months before the birth, or wait until a few months after it.
- Let your child choose some exciting new bedding for his or her "big bed". It might be easier to pick this from a catalogue rather than going to a store, which could feel intimidating.
- Put the bed where the cot used to be for familiarity.
- Get your child to help you make the bed for the first time, and ask which toys he or she wants to sleep with. Let the child keep his or her cot blanket for comfort.
- Put a guardrail on the bed to stop the child falling out.
- Praise your child for staying in a grown-up bed at night.

LOSING THE DUMMY

Lots of young children like to suck on a dummy (pacifier) for comfort. This can help to get them to sleep, but prolonged use can cause the front teeth to push forwards in some children and it may also interfere with speech development if it is used during the day. Be clear that dummies are for sleep times only. Don't let your child play or talk while sucking on a dummy.

Experts differ on when you should get rid of a dummy – some say by the child's first birthday, others by the age of three. You will have to judge when your child can lose a dummy without causing undue distress. Most children become less interested in their dummies as they grow up,

Moving into a big bed is an important transition that you want your toddler to feel good about. Don't move a child because you are having another baby and need the cot. Borrow or buy a second cot (get a new mattress) rather than oust your toddler too soon.

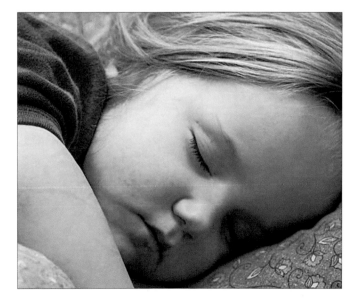

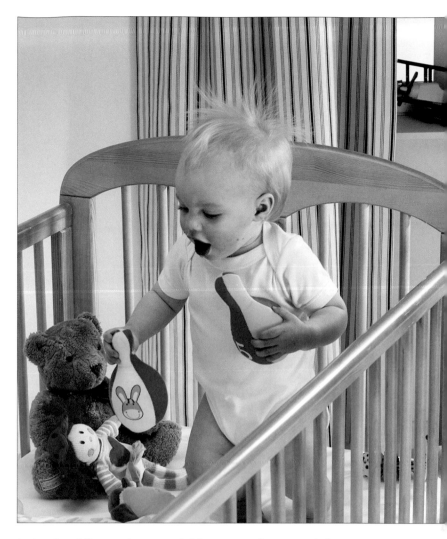

Lots of toddlers wake up at 6.00am or earlier, especially if they sleep through the night. The best solution is probably to go to bed earlier yourself. But your toddler may be happy to play for a while if you leave a different interesting toy in the cot each night.

so your child's dependence on the dummy may be lessening naturally. Try putting him or her down to sleep without it from time to time. If this works, simply offer the dummy less and less frequently.

If your child is old enough, talk about using the dummy. Say that you think he or she is now grown-up enough to stop using it. Ask your child's opinion about this. If the child is clear that he or she still wants it, let the subject drop for a while before bringing it up again. If your child is willing to consider giving up the dummy, suggest that a favourite toy can be used for comfort at night instead. A reward chart – with a sticker every time the child goes to sleep without the dummy – may help. Give lots of praise too. Don't use shame or ridicule to encourage your child to give up a dummy.

Some children benefit from ritual: a dummy fairy may come in the night and take the dummies away, leaving a gift in exchange, or your child could deposit the dummy at the dentist's in exchange for a new toothbrush.

Problems at bedtime

Some children who have slept through the night from a young age start to wake up again or resist going to bed. This is sometimes due to separation anxiety, but often it is simply down to excitement: now that your child can do so much, why would he or she want to go to bed?

BEDTIME ROUTINE

You'll find it much easier to get your child to sleep at night if you have a consistent bedtime routine. This helps a toddler to relax and get ready for sleep. Keep activities after tea gentle and quiet to help your child wind down from the day's events. It is also important to have a set bedtime – somewhere between 6.30 and 7.30 pm works well for most children, but some won't settle until later. If your child is used to a very late bedtime, bring it forwards by ten minutes a day until he or she is going to sleep at a time that works for you both.

Keep your bedtime routine short and simple – it shouldn't take longer than about half an hour. A good routine could be: playtime in the bath, getting into pyjamas, a drink of milk from a cup, toothbrushing, cuddle and storytime, then bed and lights out. Avoid doing anything upsetting at this time: if washing your

Story time is a good part of the bedtime routine, because it gives children focused time with their parent. It often becomes a treasured childhood memory.

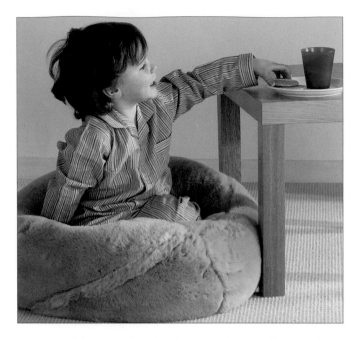

Some children need a simple snack before they go to bed. Avoid giving them anything, such as cheese or chocolate, that may affect their sleep.

child's hair makes him or her scream, do it in the morning. Resist an older toddler's attempts to extend the routine: he or she may ask you to read more stories, say, to delay bedtime. Be firm. Giving some notice of what will happen next – "After your story, it is bedtime" – will help your child to accept the inevitable.

Make sure that your child has any comforters or favourite stuffed animals that he or she needs to help get to sleep. Get a nightlight or leave a light on in the hallway if the child doesn't like to be in the dark. Some children find it comforting if you say goodnight in exactly the same way each night – for example, "Night night, darling, see you in the morning."

GETTING YOUR TODDLER TO DROP OFF ALONE

If you always stayed with your baby until he or she was asleep, your toddler is unlikely to drop off alone now. You may still be happy to stay, but you may find that going to sleep takes longer and longer. If you want your evenings to yourself – or if you have older children who need your attention as well – you will have to make a firm decision to teach your child to go to sleep without you.

Most parents find that they can improve their child's sleep within a week. But you do need to give your child a clear, consistent message about bedtime throughout this time. For this reason, you should start a sleep training

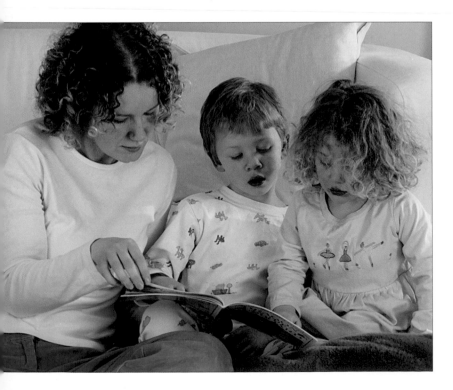

programme in a week when you will be around for every bedtime and when your child is not having to deal with any other disruptions to the normal routine, or other challenges in their life. Younger toddlers can benefit from the routines suggested for older babies, but older ones also respond very well to the kiss method.

THE KISS ROUTINE

This works best if your child is in a bed, so that you can easily bend down to kiss him or her when lying down. It could take a couple of hours and several hundred kisses if your child is very persistent. Kiss your child only when he or she is lying down, and don't be drawn into any discussion or play. Say again that you will be back in a minute to give your child another kiss, and do it as often as seems necessary.

1 Do your usual bedtime routine. Put your child to bed and give him or her a kiss goodnight.
2 Say you will be back in a minute with another kiss.
3 Turn away and then turn back and give your child a kiss straight away.
4 Move away a little further this time, then turn back and give another kiss.
5 Now do something in the room such as putting toys away or folding an item of clothing. Then turn back to your child and give another kiss.
6 Leave the room as if you are going to do something, come straight back and kiss your child again.
7 If your child gets up to follow you, act surprised and lead him or her gently back to bed. Give another kiss and then leave the room again.
8 Continue in this way for as long as it takes for your child to fall asleep. Gradually extend the period you leave between kisses.
9 Do the same on subsequent nights. You should find that it takes less time to get your child to sleep as the week draws on. But don't be surprised if you have a few setbacks: the third and fifth nights are often the worst.

THE MOVING CHAIR METHOD

An alternative method to use is the moving chair method. It can be good if your child cannot bear you to leave the room before he or she is asleep.

After your usual bedtime routine, sit on a chair beside the child's bed and turn the child so that he or she is facing away from you. Switch off the light and tell your child it is "sleepytime" (or whatever phrase you prefer to use) and to close his or her eyes. Then every time he or she tries to chat, simply say "ssshhhh, sleepytime". You will probably have to do this many times, but persevere however long it takes for your child to drop off. Over the next few nights, do exactly the same, but move the chair a little further away from the bed and towards the (open)

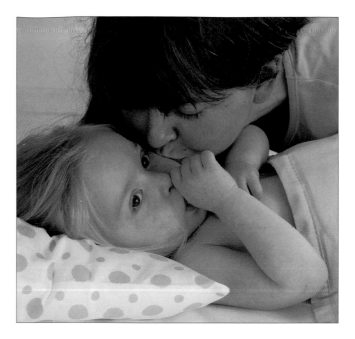

The kiss routine is a gentle way of getting your child to drop off alone, often without even realizing that that is what is happening.

door each night. Eventually you should be sitting outside the door. By this time your child should be able to drop off alone and you can leave the bedroom after you've said goodnight. Go back to sitting outside the door if he or she seems to need that reassurance for a while longer.

Help your child to see his or her bedroom as a pleasant place to be. Encourage the child to play in his or her bedroom and feel happy and relaxed in there. Don't make the bedroom a negative place by using it as a place to send older toddlers as punishment.

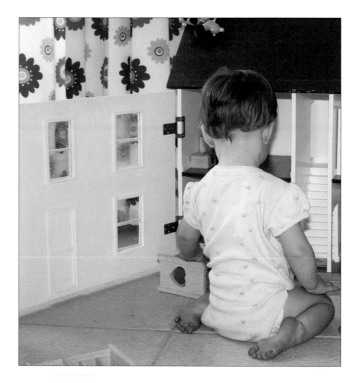

Night waking

It's hard to deal with children waking up during the night. Most of us will do anything to soothe our children so that we can get back to sleep ourselves. If your child is continually waking up and it is affecting your sleep, you probably need to steel yourself to use a sleep training technique to help him or her fall asleep without you.

It's best to start by establishing a bedtime routine first, which may resolve the problem. Give your child as few reasons as possible to get up in the night: leave a glass of water by the bedside if he or she wakes up thirsty, give the child a snack at bedtime and make sure he or she uses the toilet. If your toddler is happy to go to sleep at bedtime, but continues to wake you during the night, try to address any obvious causes first. But if your toddler simply wants your attention at night, you can do the kiss routine, controlled crying or the back-to-your-own-bed method as appropriate. As with any sleep training, you need to make a clear decision that this is what you want to do and to stick with it for a week.

WHY IS MY CHILD WAKING UP?

Night waking can have a straightforward cause and be simple to solve. Before trying any sleep training methods, consider whether your child does any of the following.

Sleeps too much during the day. Try shortening the daytime nap to one and a half hours. Don't let your child nap later than about 2.30 pm.

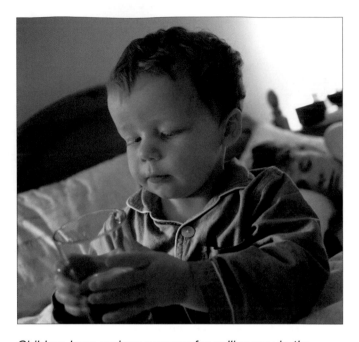

Children have various reasons for calling you in the night. Doing something as simple as leaving a glass of water in their reach can help them settle themselves.

Doesn't sleep enough during the day. Prioritize naptime. If your child won't nap, arrange some quiet time or go out for a restful journey in the buggy.

Is disturbed by outside noises. Consider moving the cot or getting thicker curtains to blot out noise. Leaving a radio set on low in the child's room helps to make outside noises less intrusive.

Is disturbed by you. Don't rush in to soothe your child; wait for a minute or two to see if he or she settles.

Gets too cold or too hot. Modify the bedding as necessary. If your child is waking from the cold when your heating goes off, add another blanket at your bedtime.

Is anxious when alone. Give lots of attention during the day and put your baby in a room with a sibling if you have other children. Consider moving your child's cot into your room, or put another bed in the child's room. When he or she wakes up, soothe your child briefly and then lie down until he or she goes back to sleep. You can then either go back to your own room or stay where you are. You can teach your toddler to sleep alone when the time is right.

Is ill or teething or has nappy (diaper) rash. Accept some broken nights as inevitable, but return to your usual routine as soon as possible.

Has night terrors or nightmares. Comfort your child immediately – don't leave him or her to cry. Put the child back to bed to sleep, but consider leaving a nightlight on.

NIGHT WAKING IN NURSING TODDLERS

Breastfeeding toddlers may continue to wake up at night to feed. If your child wakes often and you are finding it hard to function, the following may help.

- Feed more during the day. Try feeding your child in a quiet, darkened room where there are few distractions.
- Tell an older toddler that you are no longer going to feed at night – sometimes children just need to be given clear parameters.
- Ask your partner to go to your toddler at night. Your toddler is likely to protest at first, and your partner may need to be lovingly persistent in order to settle him or her. This will be easier if your partner first takes over bedtime for a few nights.
- If you are sharing a room, consider moving your child into a different room, or sleep elsewhere yourself for a few nights.

CONTROLLED CRYING FOR NIGHT WAKING

When your child cries in the night, listen to the cries. Go in straight away if you think the child is frightened or in pain. If you are sure he or she is just calling out for you, you can try this method. Remember that you can adapt it: your limit could be five minutes of crying.

1 Wait for a minute or so before you go in. Briefly check that the child's clothing isn't wet or tangled and that his or her comforter hasn't got lost. Soothe the child with a few shushes or by stroking his or her back. Don't pick your child up or linger longer than 30 seconds or so.

2 Let the child cry but go back at increasing intervals to repeat the soothing. Start with two minutes, then three, then five, then eight, then ten, then 15.

3 Keep returning at intervals of 15 minutes until the child falls asleep. If he or she wakes up again, repeat the process over again.

YOUR TODDLER AND YOUR BED

Lots of children get up in the night and come into their parents' bed. This is fine if you are happy with it, and it doesn't affect your sleep, your partner's or your child's. But you will probably find it does disturb you, and that either you or your partner ends up sleeping elsewhere while your child lies horizontally across your pillows.

If you are happy for your child to come in with you:

- Consider setting a limit to give you and your partner some privacy – for example, no toddlers in your bed before 2.00 am.
- Get a large bed that accommodates everyone.
- Put a small mattress next to your bed, and get your child to sleep there. Tell him or her to come in quietly "like a little mouse" so as not to disturb you.

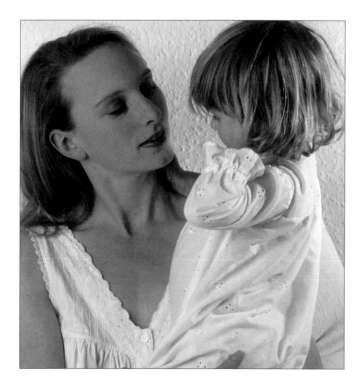

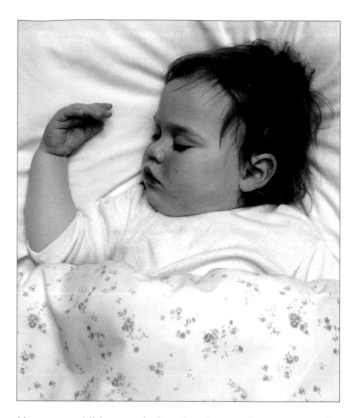

How your child naps during the day can be a cause of poor sleep at night. Think about whether he or she gets too little naptime – or too much.

The back to your own bed method:

1 When your child appears at your bedside, take him or her back to bed. Say it is bedtime, give the child a cuddle and then go back to your own bed.

2 The next time the child appears in your room, do the same thing.

3 If the child continues to appear, then gently lead him or her back to bed in silence. Do this as often as it takes until he or she stays there, even if you have to do it 30 times or more.

4 Don't get annoyed, and don't engage in any chat or explanations. Make sure your partner has the same approach: it is essential to be consistent.

After a nightmare, soothe and reassure your toddler before helping him or her get back to a peaceful sleep in his or her own bed.

NIGHT TERRORS

Some children have night terrors, in which they may scream, thrash about, sit up and look terrified for several minutes. Stay with your child while this is going on, but don't wake him or her. If the terrors tend to happen at the same time each night, try waking your child up 15 minutes beforehand and keeping him or her awake for a few minutes.

Toddler development and play

❝ You will be constantly surprised and delighted by your toddler's skills and attainments and you will bask in the reflected glory. ❞

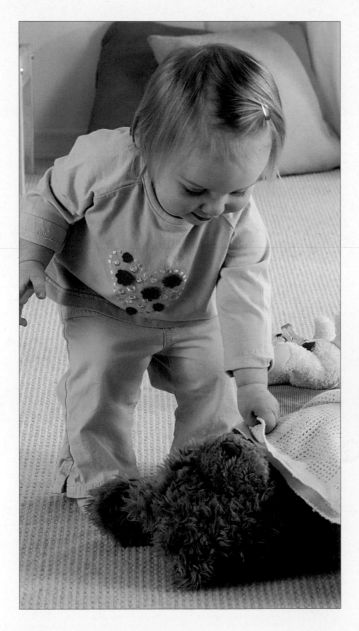

Curiosity is the defining characteristic of young toddlers. From the age of about 16 months, your child will acquire an insatiable appetite for new sights and experiences, novel words and situations, and will want to share this new knowledge with you. He or she may exclaim "Car!" every time one goes past (even if that's every two seconds as you go down the street), or may cry "Woof!" at every four-legged beast in the park, on the television screen or in the pages of a book.

The world is full of interest for toddlers and it is fascinating to watch them explore as their daring and confidence grow. You will be constantly surprised and delighted by your toddler's skills and attainments and you will bask in the reflected glory when your child succeeds in coming all the way down the stairs, sliding on his or her bottom. This is the time of walk and talk. Your child can now get out of the buggy and walk down the street with you and his or her capacity for language will suddenly race ahead at an exponential rate.

A growing emotional maturity may show itself in caring behaviour. Your child may like looking after a teddy bear or dolly, putting it to bed, "feeding" it and so on.

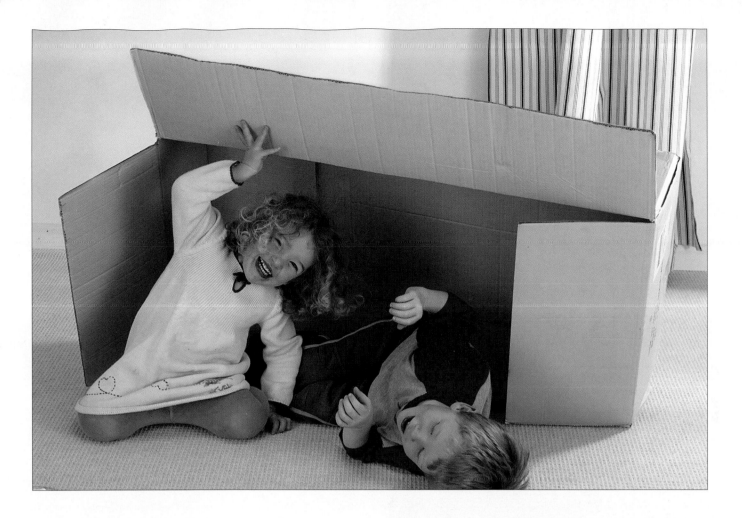

But at the start of their third year, children are in many ways still babies. Toddlers are totally concerned with themselves and do not yet understand about other people and their needs. Yet they already have views of their own about what they should be doing, and will protest loudly if adults try to make them do something they disagree with. This can be frustrating – lots of people dub this time the "terrible twos" – but it is very natural. Your toddler is learning how to be a separate, self-sufficient person. As a parent, you have the tricky job of policing and keeping your child safe, while encouraging this new-found independence and individuality. Your toddler will frustrate and exasperate you at times. But this age is also fun. Your child's emerging personality will make you proud and keep you constantly amused.

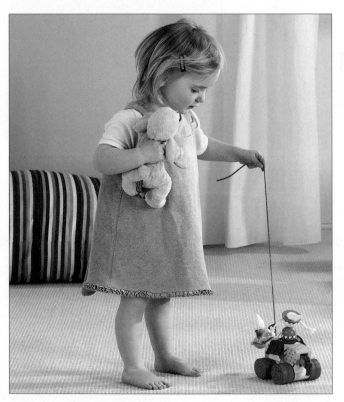

Top: Toddlers enjoy playing alongside other children from the age of about 18 months. An older child will keep your toddler happily engaged for long periods.

A treasured favourite toy may accompany a toddler everywhere for a while, even if he or she is actively playing with another toy.

First steps

Babies officially become toddlers when they learn to walk by themselves. Most children learn to walk when they are between 11 and 14 months, but some children walk as early as nine months and some can wait until 18 months. A child who isn't walking by then is probably just taking his or her time, but it is worth checking with a doctor to be on the safe side.

Your toddler will start walking as an extension of cruising. A gap between two pieces of furniture provides the impetus to take the first step: you can deliberately move them apart when you think he or she is ready to do this. Having been brave enough to take the first independent steps, your child will love to launch himself or herself from a piece of furniture towards you, or, better still, from one person to another – kneel on the floor, hold your arms out and call to him or her as encouragement. It can take several weeks before your baby gains the confidence to go further and walk across a room.

When they first start walking, toddlers rock from one foot to another, keeping their feet wide apart to help them balance. They also hold their arms away from the body for the same reason. As they gradually get steadier on their feet, they walk with the feet closer together. Your toddler will learn to bend and pick something up from the floor without losing his or her balance and will enjoy carrying

Learning walking skills starts early: a baby will enjoy supported standing from a few months old, and, once they learn to step, they will love to walk with your help.

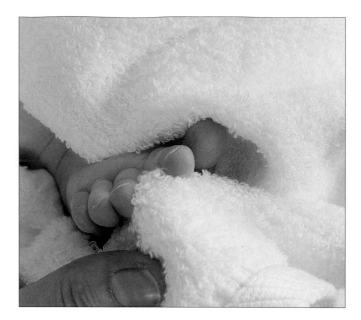

Wash your child's feet every day and dry between the toes – toddlers' feet can sweat a lot. Keep toenails trimmed, or they will press against the shoes and may become ingrowing.

something from one part of the room to another. A sturdy toddle truck will be a favourite toy, but almost anything will be pushed along the ground: a cardboard box, a chair, the buggy. As your child will now be moving more quickly than when crawling, you'll need to watch him or her closely all the time.

Once your child is good at walking, let him or her walk outside. Think of short walks you could do together rather than always using the buggy or car seat. Many parents frown on reins because they think they are restrictive, but they are a good way of giving active toddlers more freedom while keeping them safe.

WHAT SHOES?

Walking barefoot helps to strengthen the muscles in the feet, so don't put your child in shoes until he or she is ready to walk outside. Even then, let your child go barefoot indoors or just put on socks for warmth.

When you shop for shoes, it is very important that you go to a store that measures children's feet properly and offers shoes in different widths as well as lengths. The bones of a young child's foot are very soft so they can easily be damaged if they are constricted by a badly fitting shoe. Never buy shoes off the peg, and don't put your child in second-hand shoes – they will have slightly distorted to the shape of the previous wearer's feet, and

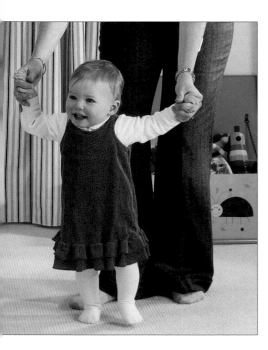

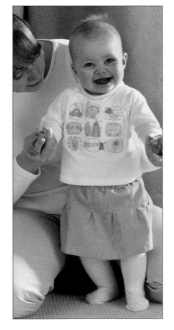

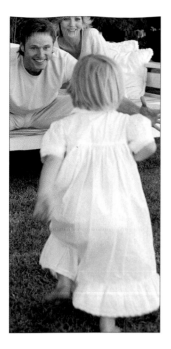

Left: The first steps are short and wobbly. But your baby will be incredibly pleased with himself or herself for managing such an awesome feat, and will be thrilled by your delight in this accomplishment.

Right: Push-along toys can help to give a new walker extra confidence. Later on, your child may pretend it is, say, a vacuum cleaner in imaginative play.

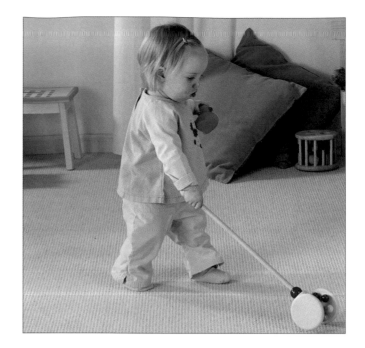

won't give proper support to your child's feet. A properly fitted shoe should have lots of "growing room" in the toe area, and the sole should be flexible, so that it moves with your child's foot. The shoe should fasten securely with a buckle, Velcro or laces. The heel of the shoe should fit securely: it shouldn't come off the heel when your child stands on tiptoes. Choose shoes made of natural materials (such as leather or canvas), which allow the foot to "breathe".

Have your child's feet measured every six to eight weeks, a good shoe shop should do this – and check that your child's shoes are still fitting properly – without putting you under any pressure to buy.

SAFETY CHECK

Your toddler will be able to stretch for things when standing up – which means he or she can get to objects that were previously out of reach. Assess your living space afresh and take steps to make it as safe as possible.

- Don't leave cutlery, cups or glasses near the edges of tables.
- Make sure that carpets and rugs are smooth: a rucked-up rug is a hazard for your uncertain walker.
- If you have a hard floor surface, don't put your child in slippy socks: he or she needs to be barefoot or should wear non-slip socks.
- If older children are playing a game nearby, move a toddler out of their way or he or she is likely to get knocked over.
- Don't allow play with lightweight toy buggies until your toddler's balance has improved to the point where he or she doesn't tip them over.

IS SOMETHING WRONG?

Toddlers walk in a different way to adults – they tend to keep their feet apart, and they "waddle" because they walk with flat feet. Normally these little oddities resolve themselves in time, but do seek medical advice if you are concerned about your child's feet or the way that he or she walks, or if any of the following conditions are severe or affect one leg only.

Pigeon toes (toeing in). Some children walk with their toes turned in. This usually corrects itself in time, but see your doctor if your child turns only one foot in or out, or if there is no improvement by the age of seven or eight.

Dancer toes (toeing out). Other children keep their toes turned outwards when they first start to walk. This usually improves within a year or so.

Flat feet. All children are flat footed when they start to walk; this gives them more stability. The arch of the foot doesn't start to develop until a child is about two, and your child won't walk with a heel-to-toe step for another year after that. If flat feet persist after age three, ask your doctor to refer your child to a podiatrist (foot specialist).

Bow legs. You'll see a gap between your child's ankles and knees until the age of about two. But if the gap is very pronounced or persists, ask a health professional to take a look – very occasionally this is a sign of rickets.

Knock knees. Lots of children hold their knees together when they walk: a gap of up to 6cm/2¾in between the ankles is normal. Knock knees usually go by age six.

SOCKS

Only buy cotton socks for your toddler and make sure that they fit properly. Tight socks can be as damaging as tight shoes.

Your young toddler's development

Six months or so after learning to walk, your toddler will start to run, but he or she will find it hard to stop or slow down to turn corners. "Chasing" a child towards a sofa that he or she can land on safely is great fun and helps to strengthen the leg muscles and improve control. Outdoor games, such as football, will help with balance – your toddler won't be able to kick a ball accurately for a while, but he or she will have a lot of fun trying.

A toddler is hardwired to practise all the movements needed to improve his or her coordination and control. A child who has balance will instinctively squat to pick something up. This builds flexibility in the hips and knees and strengthens the leg muscles. He or she will also practise walking backwards and sideways. Most young children love dancing, which gives an ideal opportunity to practise a whole range of different movements: dance together and incorporate knee bends, swaying, arm movements and different steps into your routine.

The stairs will continue to be a source of fascination. Young toddlers learn to walk up them instead of crawling, but have to bring both feet on to one step at a time, at first holding on to the step above. The next stage is to walk up without holding on, but they can't do this using alternate feet until they are about three. It's good to let

As your child's thinking ability develops, you may notice that he or she pauses before tackling a task to consider how to go about it. Shape sorters teach children about shapes and sizes and give a sense of accomplishment.

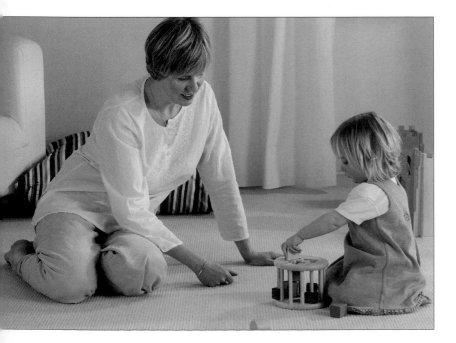

your child practise going up and down stairs, but you'll need to be close behind. A toddler is very likely to pause halfway up and, forgetting where he or she is, may lean backwards with inevitable results. Coming down is harder than going up; teach your child to do it backwards, on his or her tummy. Continue to use stair gates to prevent your child from shimmying up or down unaccompanied.

USING THE HANDS

During the second year, children learn to rotate the wrist, which allows them to be much more controlled in their hand movements. They can build a tower, placing one brick on another: by about 18 months they can manage a tower of three or four bricks, and will be able to add a couple more by the age of two. They can bring a spoon to their mouth without spilling too much food and can learn to drink from an open cup, provided they are given the opportunity.

At the same time, the small motor skills become more refined. Toddlers learn to use just a finger to point rather than involving the whole arm and hand. They can grasp a zipper tag between finger and thumb and pull it open and shut, and can twist knobs on the hi-fi. They learn to use a pencil more deliberately: by the end of the year they can make simple lines and semicircles as well as scribbles.

MENTAL LEAPS

These developing physical skills allow your child to explore the world and to get a better sense of how things work. They go hand in hand with brain development: burgeoning cognitive skills make themselves known in physical achievements, and exploration of the physical world stimulates the child's mind.

Toddlers naturally want to experiment with things, because this is how they learn about them. So they will press buttons on the washing machine, reach for door knobs, and post toast into the VCR. They will test everything – you can almost see them thinking, "What happens if I press this?", or "What does this do?"

INDIVIDUAL DEVELOPMENT
Children progress at different rates, but if you are worried at any time about any area of your child's growth and development, raise it with a health professional. You will be invited to a checkup to review your child's progress at around 18 months.

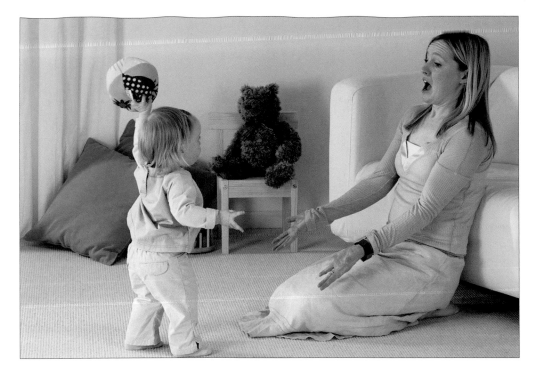

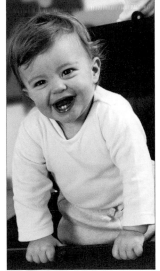

Once they've worked out how to do it, toddlers will love to make you laugh.

At some time in the second year children learn to throw overhand. Give your toddler a foam ball for safe throwing at home.

Memory steadily improves along with motor skills. Your child's new capacity to remember will show itself in play and the ability to anticipate events. If you are getting your coat to go out, your child may follow suit and go and stand by the door. If you were sweeping the floor this morning and have left the broom out, he or she may well grasp it and try to do the same in the afternoon or the next day. This is called deferred imitation.

Memory is, of course, essential for the development of language. There is a huge variation in the amount young toddlers speak, but most are able to name lots of familiar objects and to put two words together – "Mummy phone", "Louie ball", "more milk" – by the end of the second year. You will notice that your toddler's ability to understand you is way ahead of his or her ability to talk – a child will fetch a teddy when you ask for it many months before he or she says the word.

EMOTIONAL DEVELOPMENT

Your baby gradually learns that he or she is an individual, separate from you. Sometimes this feels scary and may make a child anxious and clingy. But a toddler slowly gets more comfortable with the idea. After about 18 months, he or she will be happier to spend longer periods away from you.

A growing sense of self means that a child starts to assert his or her will by refusing to do things that don't appeal – expect to hear the word "no" a lot. It can be quite sad to say goodbye to the compliant and unquestioning baby you have nurtured, but this new individualism is an essential part of growing up. Your child needs to be allowed to probe the limits of self-reliance, and will do so happily if you provide a loving, stable base to return to. Now, when you go to a parent-and-toddler group, your child will venture farther away from you, returning from time to time for reassurance that you are still there.

Although your toddler's behaviour is bound to test you at times, you'll notice a burgeoning awareness of other people that marks the start of socialization. This starts with you: your child will know when you are sad, for example, and will grasp which aspects of his or her behaviour please or displease you.

During his or her second year, a young child will find it easier to grasp a pencil and make marks.

Children are fascinated by zips, and work out how to manipulate them by about 18 months.

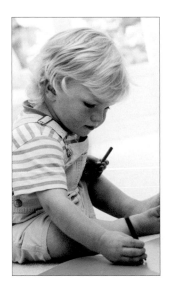

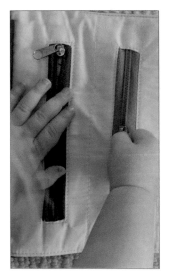

Your older toddler's development

Older toddlers are on the move all the time and they naturally have a lot more physical confidence than younger ones. Their improved sense of equilibrium means that by the age of two and a half they are proficient runners. By the end of the year they can jump off a step. They may also be able to stand on one leg for a few seconds, though they have to concentrate hard. They can kick and throw with much greater accuracy, throwing underarm as well as overarm, and they may be able to catch a ball (though they still miss more often than not).

CLIMBING CONFIDENCE

Older toddlers are much better at climbing, but how high your child climbs will depend on his or her individual sense of adventure. A child who is a natural risk taker may joyfully scramble up a climbing frame or on to a proper chair without considering how he or she is going to get down again. If this is the case, you will need to set limits. If your child is physically timid, he or she may be fearful of climbing. It may help your child to gain confidence if you encourage some practice on manageable pieces of play equipment, such as the first few rungs of the slide ladder, while you stand behind him or her.

If you have stairs in your home, your toddler will by now have had lots of practice at negotiating them. By the age of three, a child may walk up a flight of stairs as adults do, putting alternate feet on the steps. Coming down is trickier, and your child may continue to bring both feet on to each step until around four. If your home is on one level, then you might want to use a friend's home to get your child accustomed to negotiating stairs safely.

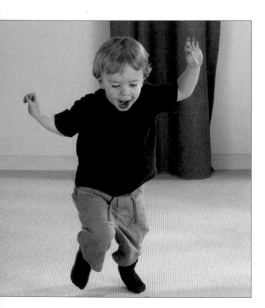

Jumping develops slowly. Most 18-month-olds can't manage to bend their knees and get themselves off the ground at the same time, but they may manage this feat by the age of two. Hopping comes much later.

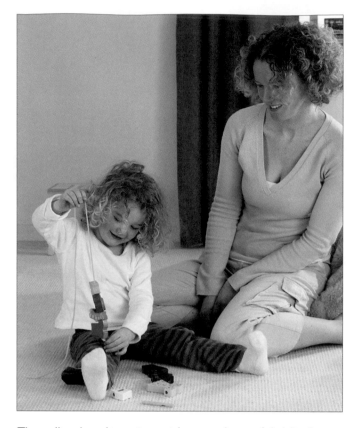

Threading beads on to a string requires a fair bit of manual dexterity. This toy is also great for counting games and learning the names of colours.

USING THE HANDS

At two, children can turn over one page of a book at a time, rather than two or three. They can also thread beads on to a string, provided the holes are large enough. And towers of bricks get higher: they can manage up to eight blocks by the age of two and a half. As children's hand movements continue to become more precise, they are able to tackle more everyday tasks: for example, doing up large buttons or toggles. Get your child to help you with jobs such as setting the table. Tackling everyday tasks will help his or her dexterity and build self-confidence.

Your child will have a lot more control when using a pencil or crayon: he or she won't be able to draw a

RIGHT- AND LEFT-HANDEDNESS
Lots of children are ambidextrous until the age of three. But you may notice that your child shows a definite preference for using the right or left hand when eating or playing.

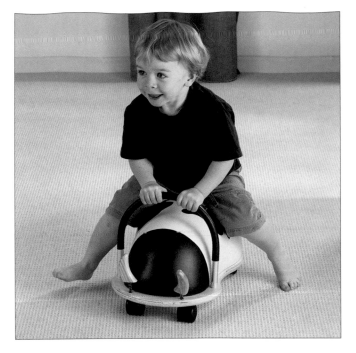

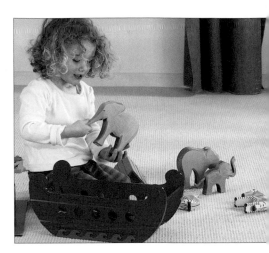

picture yet, but will do lots of lines, dots and circles. By the end of the year, your child can probably manage a pair of children's safety scissors (supervised by you), though only to cut simple strips rather than complicated outlines at first. Using scissors is a complex manoeuvre, involving forethought, dexterity and concentration. Your toddler will have taken a big step forward when he or she can manipulate a pair of scissors.

MENTAL LEAPS

Your toddler has now garnered enough knowledge about how things work to be able to organize and sort things: he or she may place bricks in a line, say, or put toy animals in one box and toy cars in another. Older toddlers are able to "think" about things that aren't right in front of them, which means they can be much more imaginative in play. Now your child doesn't necessarily need a toy as inspiration – he or she is able to pretend that a cardboard box, say, is a car or a house. In the toddler's make-believe world, ideas are drawn from everything – the daily routine, the people he or she knows, television shows and story

books. Your child's memory has improved to the extent that if you interrupt in the middle of a game, the child will be able to return to it and pick up where he or she left off. Language skills are developing rapidly and he or she will probably be talking in simple sentences by the age of three. You'll also see your toddler playing sorting games with toys, showing the natural urge to classify and categorize that is a very important skill for life: to function in the world, we need to be able to tell what's hot from what's cold, who is friendly and who is not, what is ours and what is someone else's.

EMOTIONAL DEVELOPMENT

During their third year, children develop a much better sense of the world and their place within it. Until now they have seen everything in relation to themselves. Now they start to realize that other people have needs, too. They also become more affectionate.

Toddlers develop a much stronger sense of self from about two years. This goes hand-in-hand with a new possessiveness. Another important part of the sense of self is an awareness of gender. This starts as early as 18 months, and children are sure in the knowledge that they are boys or girls by the age of three. They may start to behave in stereotypical ways at this point, particularly if they feel that this is what is expected of them.

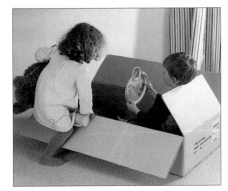

Who needs expensive toys when a large cardboard box can be a car...

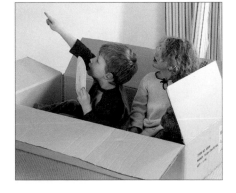

... a spaceship navigating the universe of the living room...

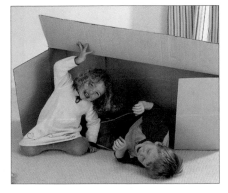

... or a special den in which to hide away from the grown-ups?

An expanding family

Young children love stability and routine, but they inevitably have to deal with change and new challenges from time to time. Probably the biggest upheaval of a child's early life is the arrival of a baby brother or sister, and sensitive handling is necessary to help a toddler accept a new baby.

PREPARING FOR A NEW BABY

Pack away any of your child's baby gear long before the arrival of the new baby. That way, your toddler is less likely to feel that the baby is taking things that belong to him or her when you get them out again. The toddler will also enjoy looking at them all again and helping you decide which toys to put out for the new baby.

Tell your child that you have a baby in your tummy once you start getting large – before other people let it slip. Older children may like to feel the baby kick or to listen to its heartbeat at your antenatal checkups. But ultrasound pictures can look bizarre, so don't show the scan unless you think your child is up to it.

Introducing a second child into your family can have its tricky moments, but your oldest will learn to accept his or her sibling in time.

WEANING A TODDLER

If you are still breastfeeding your toddler when you become pregnant, it is fine to continue. Some mothers decide to feed both their newborn and toddler at the same time (tandem feeding). However, if you decide to wean your toddler before the birth, it is best to start several months beforehand. The most natural way to wean is using the principle of "never offer, never refuse": nurse your toddler if he or she asks, but don't offer a feed. This can work well for some children, but you may also need to do the following as well.

• Give your child a drink and a snack before your usual nursing times.
• Think about when your child likes to nurse. Change your routine so that he or she will naturally ask to nurse less often.
• If your child nurses irregularly, try postponing the feed and then provide a distraction by going out together or playing a game.
• If you usually feed on waking and at bedtime, get the child's dad or someone else to take over at these times.

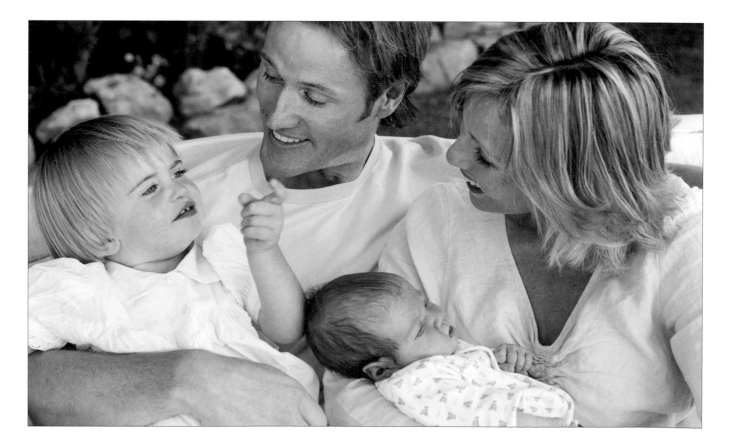

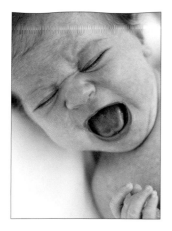

Left: Looking after a new baby and a toddler is hard work, so make sure you get enough rest.

Right: Encourage an older child to play nicely with a new baby and exclaim at how the baby seems to like him or her the most.

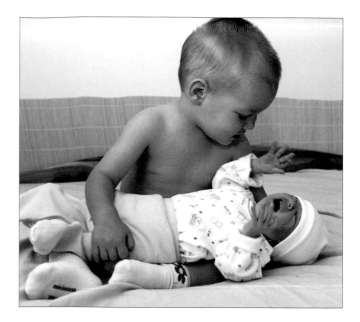

Don't make any major changes to your child's routine near the delivery date. Potty training, or moving a toddler to his or her own room or into a proper bed, should happen either a few months before the birth or once the child has got used to the new baby.

Talk to your child about what life will be like when the baby comes. It can help to reminisce about his or her own babyhood: tell stories about how your toddler kept you up all night. Give your child the opportunity to ask questions and voice any concerns, and be honest but reassuring in your answers – for example, agree that things will be different when the new baby comes, but talk about all the things that will stay the same too. If you have friends with small babies, it is a good idea to take your child with you to visit them. If possible, let him or her see other mothers breastfeeding and explain what is happening.

Let your toddler know who will care for him or her while you have the baby. It is much better to get a familiar person to come to your home rather than sending your child to stay with someone. However, if he or she has to go and stay elsewhere, be sure to arrange a couple of practice runs before the birth. If you plan to have the baby at home, you will still need a trusted person to care for your child. Childbirth is intense and messy, even when it is going well: you will need all your energy to focus on your contractions, and your child could be traumatized by witnessing his or her mummy in labour.

INTRODUCING A NEW SIBLING

After the birth, have your arms free for hugs when you see your child for the first time – put the baby in a cot or basket for a while. Tell your toddler how much you've missed him or her. If you are coming home from hospital, get someone else to carry the new baby into your home so that you can give your full attention to your older child. Look at the baby together. Children often find small babies fascinating, and your toddler may enjoy examining the funny squashed-up face or tiny wrinkly fingers with you. Let the toddler stroke the baby gently, and say how much the baby likes it; show your child how the baby will grip his or her finger to say hello.

Give your older child a small gift "from the baby". You can put this at the foot of the baby's cot for your child to discover. You may also like to give a gift from Mummy and Daddy at some point over the next few days – a present can be a tangible reminder of how much you love your child. For an older child, it can be helpful to choose a gift that subtly reaffirms his or her place in the home, such as a new duvet cover or a special cup. Remind grandparents and close friends to say hello to your older child before cooing over the newborn. If they are bringing a gift for the baby, suggest it would be good if they brought something small for the older child as well.

AS TIME GOES ON

Emphasize how lucky the baby is to have your older child as a sibling, rather than how nice it is for the toddler to have a playmate. Try not to go on too much about the "big brother/sister" role – your child doesn't want to be seen as an adjunct to the new baby, and don't expect your child to feel instant love for your new baby. Help him or her enjoy the strangeness of the new baby instead – have a joke about the stinky nappies, the baby's funny little sneezes and yawns. Your child is bound to feel jealous of the new baby from time to time. Acknowledge this feeling and reaffirm how much you love him or her, but be firm that any rough behaviour around the baby is not to be tolerated.

Make the baby's feeding time a special time for your older child too – you can read stories, chat, do a jigsaw or listen to a story tape together while feeding. Let your older child help you care for the baby by fetching nappies or pushing the buggy, and praise him or her for helping.

Stick to your normal routines – bedtime, mealtimes and so on – as much as possible. Spend some time alone with your older child if you can: ideally, go on one outing a week while a grandparent or your partner babysits. Choose something you have always done together.

Helping toddlers play

It is during toddlerhood that children learn to learn: patterns acquired now will stay with them into their school years. But don't feel that you have to hothouse them with endless classes, planned activities and flash cards – too much structured time can be tiring for your child and doesn't leave enough time for imaginative play.

Your child will learn best in a stimulating and loving environment, with plenty of time for unhurried, self-directed play. Play will teach your toddler all he or she needs to know about problem solving, making judgements, being creative, gaining self-confidence, taking risks, developing empathy and – eventually – sharing. Here are some ways to help a toddler enjoy play.

Give your child your undivided attention when you play with him or her. Sit on the floor and do what the child wants. There's no substitute for one-on-one time, and play helps to build a good relationship.

Have fun together. Play is supposed to be enjoyable, and your child will love it if you introduce an element of humour into games.

Follow your child's lead. If your child is playing a game of make-believe, then do what he or she asks you – don't say how things ought to be. If your child needs your help to build a castle, let him or her be the architect and decide which brick goes where. Being in charge of the game helps to boost your child's self-confidence and encourages problem solving.

Don't interfere if your child is playing happily. Wait until he or she needs or asks for your input, and don't interfere or make suggestions.

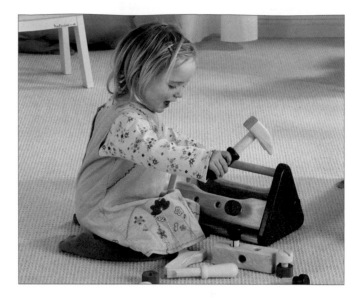

Construction toys are lots of fun, and a kit like this will cover several months of your toddler's development.

> **BALANCING A CHILD'S PERSONALITY TRAITS**
> By the time your child is two you may have a clear idea of his or her personality. Your child needs to be loved for who he or she is, but you can still use playtime constructively. If your child can't concentrate for long, for example, help by choosing an activity that he or she enjoys and then praising the child for sticking with it. Look out for the moment when the child gets bored and alter the activity slightly to reignite his or her interest.

Children are often interested in counting at an early age. They may be quick to recognize numbers long before they understand what they are for.

Rough and tumble is good for children, so long as they are enjoying it. It can help to make girls more physically confident and can help boys to manage aggression.

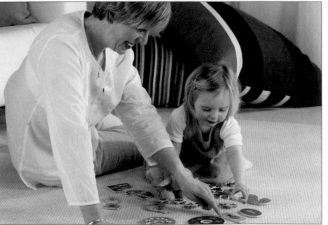

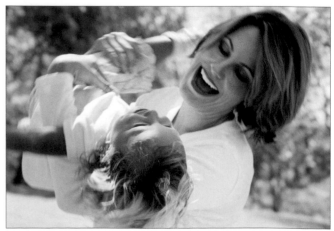

TODDLERS AND TELEVISION

Television has a mesmerizing effect, so it is tempting to allow your child to watch it when you need a break. But watching a lot of television on a regular basis can affect a toddler's ability to concentrate. A study by the American Academy of Pediatrics found that the likelihood of a child developing attention problems at school went up by 10 per cent for every hour of television watched each day – so a child watching three hours a day was 30 per cent more likely to have attention deficit disorder (ADD) by the age of seven. Excessive television at an early age has also been linked to obesity and aggression.

- Don't put a child under two in front of the television. Many children this age won't be interested in watching anyway.
- Limit older toddlers to 30 minutes at a time.
- Choose your child's viewing carefully. Children's programmes often have an educational theme and most children prefer them to adult programmes.
- Be wary of allowing your child to see advertisements. Watch videos instead of commercial programmes.
- Stay with your older toddler while he or she watches a programme and talk about it afterwards.
- Never have the television on in the background while your child is playing.

YOUR CHILD'S TOYS

Toys are more inviting if they are organized than if they are piled in a messy heap. Make tidying up part of play – your child can have just as much fun putting toys back in the box as emptying it. It's a good idea to rotate toys: if you put some away in a cupboard for a while your child will be much more interested in them when they reappear.

Provide some creative play materials, such as play dough or clay, paints, craft materials and dressing-up clothes. Let your child play with natural materials, such as snow, sand, water, mud and grass, as much as possible. Don't feel that you need to invest in electronic

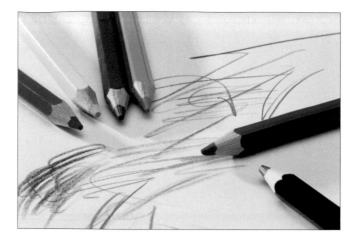

Making marks on paper is something that most children love to do, and it is an important precursor of writing, so keep chunky pencils, crayons and paper at hand.

"educational" toys. High-tech toys are very appealing to young children, but flashing lights and robotic sounds offer less potential for creative play than simple toys and play materials.

Encourage your child to play with a wide range of toys, including those aimed at the opposite gender. Different toys encourage different skills, so limiting your child early on could discourage some aspects of development: for example, playing with dolls can help with social skills, while using construction blocks helps with visual-spatial skills. Look for books that show, say, girls being brave and boys being sensitive to help your child get a broad understanding of how boys and girls behave.

It is important that your child's toys and books should accurately represent his or her world. For example, most dolls are based on Caucasian people, so if you are black or Asian, seek out toys that reflect your skin colour and make sure your child has books that feature people of your ethnic group. Studies show children can become aware of differences in skin colour by the age of two.

If you need to get on with other things, make sure your toddler has something fun to do. But don't expect your child to stay occupied for long periods.

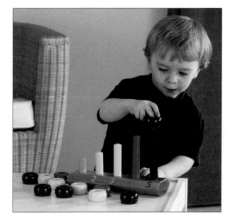
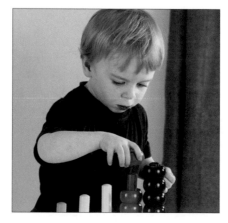
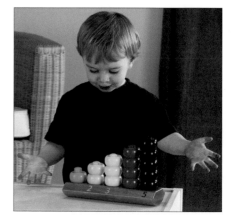

Ideas for play

Give your child a good balance of different forms of play. Toddlers need plenty of running around to let off steam, but they also need quiet activities such as looking at books or playing with bricks to help build concentration. Here are some ideas.

PHYSICAL PLAY

Toddlers have boundless energy, so give them lots of opportunity to expend it. You'll find a toddler easier to manage if he or she gets plenty of physical activity. Spend time outdoors every day if you can. Go to the park, where your child can run, jump and climb. Take your child to the local swimming pool or to a toddler gym (soft room) or go to a dancing class for older toddlers. Take short walks together and point out things that you see, hear or smell – the more children use their senses, the more they learn. On windy days, give an older toddler a length of ribbon and get the child to run so that it streams behind him or her. Some small children take a lively interest in the wildlife that can be found in a garden or park – the woodlice, worms, birds and spiders. You can foster this interest by feeding the ducks or visiting farms and zoos.

If you are stuck indoors with a fidgety toddler, push the furniture out of the way and have a mini-exercise class: touch toes, do star jumps (jumping with legs and arms wide open), run, hop, jump, spin around. Dance to some fast music: your two year old may well have a favourite tune you can dance to. Make a mini-obstacle course: create a tunnel out of a couple of chairs and a blanket, put down large open boxes for your child to crawl through and make a mountain of pillows to climb. For a calming down activity, try doing a few simple yoga poses.

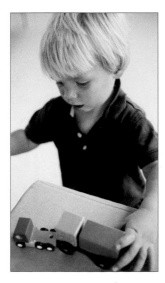

Once children develop the ability to play imaginatively, they can amuse themselves for much longer. A railway set or garage with toy cars will provide fun for many years to come as your child's play adapts to his or her growing abilities.

MAKE YOUR OWN PLAY DOUGH

Toddlers love playing with dough and it's easy to make your own. The dough will last a month or so if you store it in an airtight box in the refrigerator.

250g/8oz water
250g/8oz plain flour
30ml/2 tbsp cream of tartar
a few drops of food colouring
15ml/1 tbsp sunflower or other cooking oil
125g/4oz salt

Put all the ingredients in a small saucepan, place over a medium heat and stir until the mixture forms a smooth dough. Remove from the pan and leave to cool before using.

MESSY PLAY

Making a mess is tremendous fun, teaches your child about textures and encourages free expression. Make it a rule that your child covers up with an apron or similar (an older child's shirt, worn back-to-front, works well) and lay newspaper over the table or floor if you are using paints.
Water. Fill a washing-up bowl with water and let your child play with it, supervised, in the garden. Old yoghurt pots, bottles, straws, a funnel, spoons and a colander are all good to play with. If you have a patio, give your child a paintbrush for "drawing" on the paving, or show him or her how to step in the water and make wet footprints.
Sand. Fill a washing-up bowl with clean sand. Show your child how to make patterns in it. Provide a small jug of water to wet the sand so that your child can build mountains, make "cakes" and so on.
Painting. Younger toddlers can paint with their fingers, pieces of sponge, corks, cotton reels or potato printers. Give your child one colour to start with, and then another so that he or she can see what happens when the two are mixed. Your child may also like to do handprints (which make great cards for relatives). Use non-toxic finger paints or powder paints mixed with water and washing-up liquid (to make them thicker and easier to manage). Two year olds may be able to manage a chunky brush (or chunky non-toxic felt-tip pens).

DRESSING UP

Children enjoy dressing up from about 18 months. Make a collection of items from your own and your friends' or relatives' wardrobes and put them in a special dressing-up box, which you can bring out as a treat or on a rainy afternoon. Hats are good; other favoured items are sunglasses, short strings of beads, bracelets and other jewellery (check for safety), old handbags or briefcases, short nightdresses (for princess outfits), old jackets, gloves, boots, shawls and even odd lengths of glittering or shiny fabric.

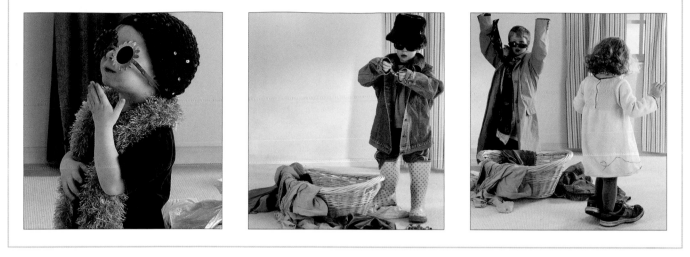

Sticking. You'll need a non-toxic glue pen, plus some small pieces of paper snipped from a magazine, bits of string, wool, ribbon and foil, dried leaves, crumpled tissues, scraps of fabric or cotton wool (cotton balls). Lentils, seeds, dried pasta shapes, loose tea leaves or desiccated coconut can all be shaken on to glued paper.

Model making. This is great fun for older toddlers. You can use all kinds of packaging: cardboard rolls, egg boxes, cereal boxes, corks, yoghurt pots and so on.

IMAGINATIVE PLAY

Toddlers have a natural instinct for copying and love pretend play. It helps them to understand their world and encourages them to use their imaginations.

Domestic play. Pretending to do chores will be a favourite game for several years. Include your child in everyday tasks when you can, such as dusting, watering plants or "cooking". Having a little helper may slow you down, but makes housework more fun. Most household items will be too heavy for your child to play with so you may want to invest in some toy domestic items.

Small world toys. Farmyards, dolls' houses, train sets, garages and so on will give your child hours of fun. Small toddlers will sort the items into groups; older ones may start to role-play with them.

Dolls and soft toys. These will be co-opted into pretend play – and may be assigned the role of a naughty toddler. Don't be surprised if they get shouted at and hit: this is how children act out aggression and difficult feelings.

To make a potato printer, cut a potato in half and use a sharp knife to trace a shape into the cut face – simple shapes work best. Cut round the shape from the side and remove the unwanted pieces. Dip the shape into paint and use as a stamp.

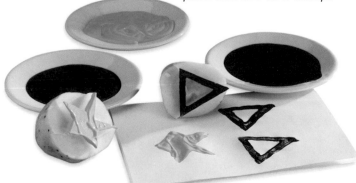

Nearly fill small plastic bottles with sand and screw the lids on tight to make skittles; arrange them in a corridor and take turns to knock them over with a soft ball.

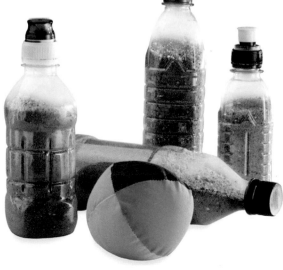

Learning to socialize

Your child's world expands gradually. As a baby, he or she was most interested in you and one or two other important people. Little by little, with your encouragement, your child has learned to interact with people such as relatives, friends, visitors and friendly passers-by. All children need to learn how to get on with other people. It's good to get your child used to being around different grown-ups and other children. This allows a toddler to get used to the idea that not everything revolves around him or her, and encourages the development of empathy, kindness and cooperation.

Most children become more sociable between the ages of 18 months and three years. But they vary greatly in how willing they are to engage with other people. Let your child develop at his or her own pace.

WHEN CHILDREN MAKE FRIENDS

Babies show interest in other children early on, but they don't know how to build relationships with each other. When your baby stretched out a hand to touch another baby's face, he or she was exploring it as much as trying to make friends.

Toddlers often respond to overtures from fun adults or older children. If your toddler has an older sibling or sees another older child regularly, the screams of delighted

Once children work out that it is more fun to play with a friend than alone, they naturally start to exhibit more cooperative and friendly behaviour.

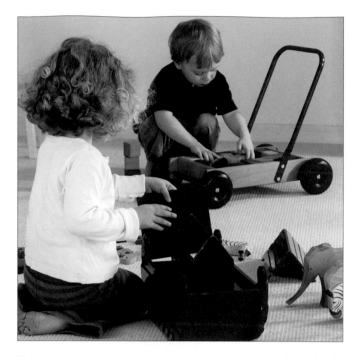

Toddlers enjoy each other's company, even if they don't play together. They may walk side by side, or sit next to each other playing with different toys. The natural instinct to be with people of the same age develops into more collaborative behaviour over time.

anticipation may show just how pleased he or she is to know them. But toddlers don't really engage with children of their own age until they are over two. They start to enjoy each other's company from about 18 months, but at

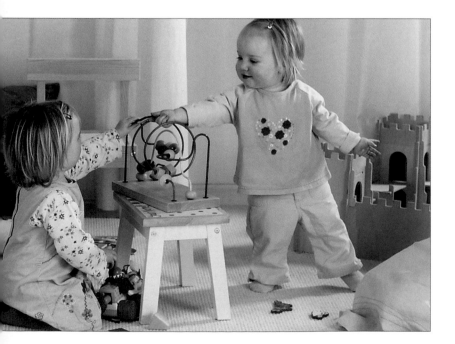

HELPING A SHY TODDLER
Some children are naturally shy and need gentle encouragement to socialize.
- Don't label your child "shy" or talk about your child's shyness in his or her hearing.
- Keep social events manageable – tea at a friend's house, a small music group.
- Give your child lots of cuddles to help him or her feel secure. But don't withdraw from the group into a corner together.
- Hold your child when a visitor arrives. Ask the child to say "hello" or wave and give lots of praise if he or she manages it.
- Look for ways to build your child's confidence: increase activities that he or she enjoys and give lots of attention and praise.

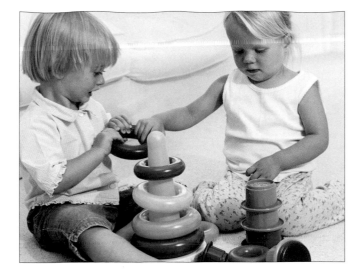

It's good to play games that involve rules or encompass turn-taking. Spell it out – say "Now it's Joe's turn", "Now it's Imogen's turn" – to drive home the message.

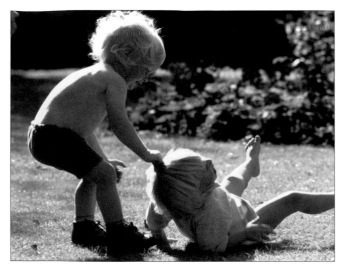

Violent outbursts are very common and need to be dealt with calmly and promptly. If your child is doing this often, you need to stick close by to pre-empt attacks.

this point they tend to play alongside each other rather than with each other (this is called parallel play). They are drawn more by the activity on offer than their liking for a particular child.

Young children are completely self-orientated. They are not aware that other people have feelings, so don't expect them to share their toys or to recognize another child's possessions: if your young toddler wants a toy, he or she will just snatch it from a companion.

BUILDING SOCIAL SKILLS

It is not until they are about three that toddlers will choose to play with a particular child, regardless of the activity. By this age, children have started to realize that other people have feelings and needs of their own. As a result, they may start to demonstrate some cooperative and considerate behaviour when playing. But playing nicely is a skill that takes time to acquire: a three year old is at the start of this process and won't be very good at it yet.

Adult supervision is still necessary to ensure that the play experience is a pleasant one for everyone. Don't leave toddlers to play on their own; you need to show them how to play together and be within earshot and visual contact to step in when conflict arises.

Encourage turn-taking. Tell one child that he or she can play with, say, the shape sorter for a little while and then it will be the other child's turn. To reinforce this (difficult) message, play games that involve taking turns or being "out".

Have clear rules. For example, say there must be no snatching or hitting. Be on the lookout for warning signs – if you can see that one child is about to take another's toy, intervene beforehand. Say, "Joe, you seem to want Mike's car. He's playing with that one, but let's see if we can find you a car too."

Avoid conflict. If other children are coming to your home, put away any toys that are particularly important to your child (older toddlers can choose which ones to put away). For older toddlers, it's helpful to introduce some activities that the children can do alongside one another, such as helping make biscuits or drawing with crayons.

Praise children for cooperative behaviour. Tell them how kind they are if they give another child a toy to play with or let another child have the first go on the slide.

Be a good role model. If you speak politely to other people, you are showing your toddler how to behave.

TRICKY BEHAVIOUR

Most toddlers lash out at other children from time to time – biting, hitting, kicking, pulling hair and so on. Like tantrums, this behaviour is mostly due to their inability to express their feelings, and it is a surefire way to get your attention. If your child hits out at another child:

- Remove your child swiftly from the situation.
- Make eye contact and tell your child in a firm voice that this behaviour is unacceptable – for example, "No biting. Biting is wrong."
- If possible, turn back to the injured party and give him or her lots of attention. But welcome your own child back with a hug quite soon.
- Never inflict the same behaviour on your child as a means of demonstrating why it is wrong. This merely sends the confusing message that biting, say, is in fact acceptable after all.
- Remember to give lots of praise when your child is playing nicely.
- Acknowledge the other parent/carer and say sorry. Even though most children hit out at some point, it is hard to see your own child hurt – a simple apology can smooth over any upset.

Talk time

Nothing is more natural than speaking. Children learn language simply by being around people who talk to them and to each other. The current thinking is that the ability to speak and understand speech is imprinted on the brain. In other words, all toddlers have an instinct for language. They recognize it for what it is and acquire it without the need to be taught. More than this, they begin to generate sentences and coin words of their own almost as soon as they learn to speak: a child may, entirely spontaneously, dub two grandmothers "Nanny-one-cat" and "Nanny-two-cats" to distinguish them. This is proof that children learn not merely by copying what they hear: they are born with an ability to make sense of the pops, hisses, grunts and whistles that make up human speech.

LANGUAGE MILESTONES

Your child is likely to say his or her first word at around one year old. The first words are usually naming words, but some children learn expressions such as "Oops" or "Oh dear" first. The words will be unclear, and may not be understood by anyone outside the family: children often

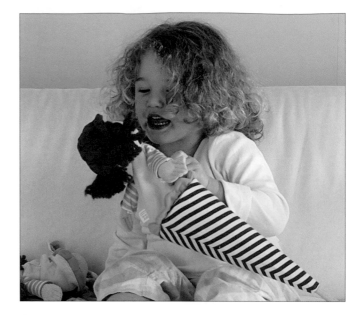

Children may start to use language in play from the age of about 18 months, and as they grow older will act out stories using conversation and dialogue.

just say the first or last consonant of a word such as "ca" for "car" or "guh" for "dog". New words are added very slowly, perhaps just one or two a month at first. But you may notice that your toddler uses the same word to mean different things and varies his or her intonation to communicate more effectively – for example, putting a rising inflection on "do-og?" to indicate a question.

By about 18 months, toddlers can understand many words: they can point out a variety of things in books and in their surroundings, they know the names of key people and understand lots of what you say. But their active vocabulary – the words they say – is likely to be around ten words. Language learning often happens in fits and starts, and children may learn lots of new words in the second six months of the year. By the age of two, they can be using 30–50 words regularly: "mine" and "no" are two favourites. They also discover how to put words together to communicate better. Most children start to say two-word sentences by the age of two – this is called "telegraphic speech".

In the third year, the use of language becomes much more sophisticated: children can tell stories, chant nursery rhymes and little songs and hold a conversation. "Why?" will soon become your child's favourite way of prolonging conversations. At three, children's vocabulary may consist of well over 300 words (some may know up to 1,000 different words by this age). They can string

---

BOOKS

Sharing books is a wonderful way of introducing new words and helping your child to understand more about the world. For younger toddlers, choose board books featuring children doing everyday things (going to bed, eating, playing) or animals. For older toddlers, choose books about counting, colours, shapes and sizes. Older toddlers will like books with simple stories or rhymes they can memorize.

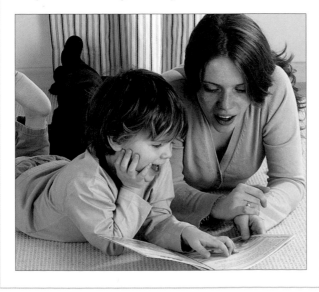

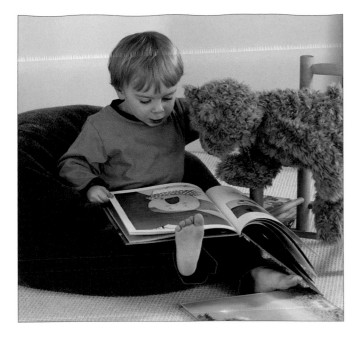

Leave books on a low shelf that your child can reach: you may be surprised at how often he or she chooses a book rather than a more active toy.

three, four or more words together in simple sentences: "Mummy go work now." They may start to use pronouns ("I", "you") as well as connecting words such as "and" and "but". Their pronunciation is clear enough to enable strangers as well as family members to understand them most of the time. They have become, in other words, social beings, able to express themselves and contribute their thoughts to society at large.

DELAYED SPEECH

The pace of language acquisition varies widely. Girls tend to speak earlier and use more words than boys, sociable toddlers talk more than shy ones and younger children in large families tend to acquire language more slowly than only or oldest children. Twins commonly experience delays in their language development: they may develop their own language, or one twin may talk for the other. It is quite possible for an intelligent child to say very little by

TWO LANGUAGES

Bilingual children learn as quickly as monolingual ones, but they may start by speaking a strange amalgam of both languages – picking and choosing words from each. It may seem that they are acquiring English more slowly than their contemporaries at first, but if this happens they will usually catch up by the age of two. Bilingualism never means that a child grows up less proficient in the language of his or her home country, and a native speaker's knowledge of more than one tongue will be a lifelong advantage.

the age of two, and language development often occurs in spurts. But if you suspect that your child's language abilities aren't progressing as they should, then do talk to a health professional. Your child can be referred to a speech therapist if necessary.

ENCOURAGING LANGUAGE

You don't need to "teach" your child to speak, but you can certainly encourage language development.

Talk lots. Studies show that children who are spoken to a lot when they are young have better vocabularies and higher IQs. Talk about what you or your child are doing. When you are out and about, point out things of interest: the red bus, the noisy pigeons and so on. If you have twins, be sure to address them individually.

Listen carefully. Toddlers' pronunciation is indistinct, so you have to concentrate to understand what they are saying. Repeating back what your child says or expanding on it shows that you are listening.

Don't answer for your child. If you ask your child a question, give him or her enough time to respond rather than jumping in. Don't finish your toddler's sentences.

Have fun with word play. Children love songs, nursery rhymes and finger games such as "Round and round the garden" and "This little piggy".

Talk about feelings. Being able to name his or her feelings will help your child to cope with them. Say things like, "Did you feel cross when I took your pencil away?" and "You have a big smile, are you feeling happy?"

If you talk to your child a lot about what he or she is doing or can see, you will naturally introduce useful new words. Older toddlers love counting games: count their toy animals, cars, socks and so on.

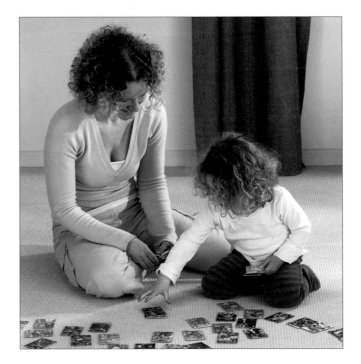

The preschool years

❝ It is important to nurture your child's self-esteem, celebrate what is special and help him or her cope with things that they find difficult. ❞

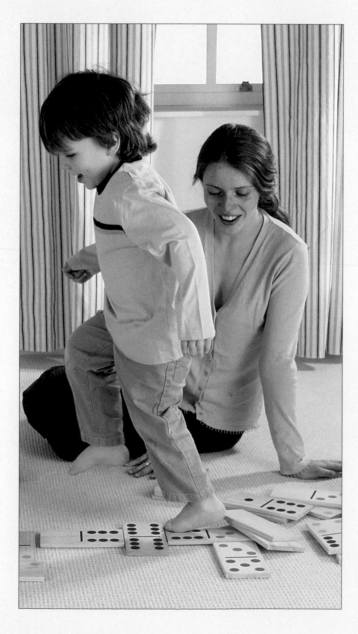

A toddler has very few social graces: when it comes to understanding the needs of other people, he or she is more like a baby than a mini-adult. But, very slowly, he or she starts to blossom into a more reasonable and social little being – someone who can think about other people. From the age of three, toddlers shows the first signs of empathy. He or she is open to persuasion, and any temper tantrums become less frequent.

A four-year-old realizes that people have feelings that must be respected, and is able to initiate friendships. He or she will share toys, invent games of their own, play for extended periods, and develop favourite pastimes. Preschool children become more aware of the differences between themselves and other people and will start to compare themselves to others. Succeeding or failing, and winning or losing all become more important issues at this stage, and it is important to nurture your child's self-esteem, celebrate what is special and help him or her to cope with things that they find difficult.

Preschool children will still have sudden mood swings, but generally will begin to become more rational and easier to negotiate with.

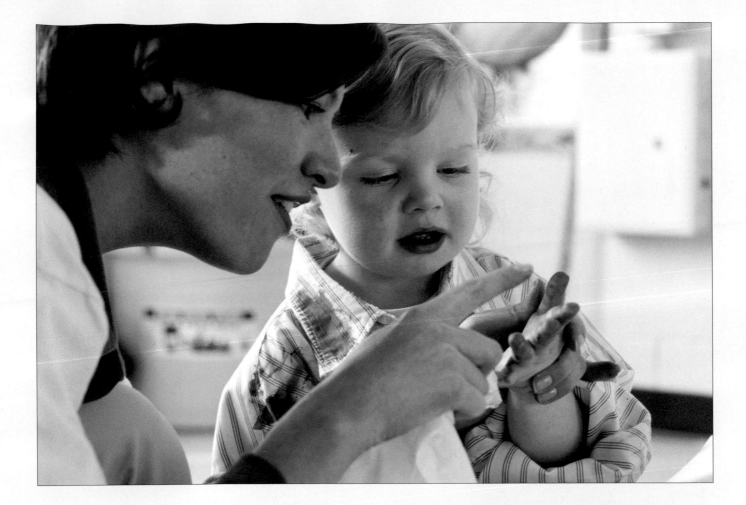

Young children love to learn, and now they have the language skills to help them. These years are a good preparation for the time when your child goes to school. Even the first term at school is a far more structured environment than your child has been accustomed to, so it is not surprising that many children get extremely tired in their first weeks and months in a school-day routine.

Good sleeping habits and a healthy diet, established over these early years, will help your child to cope. Your child will also get a new sense of himself or herself as a member of a group. Mixing with other children in the preschool years helps with this process, and all that play will have given him or her a love of learning that will help in the first steps of formal education.

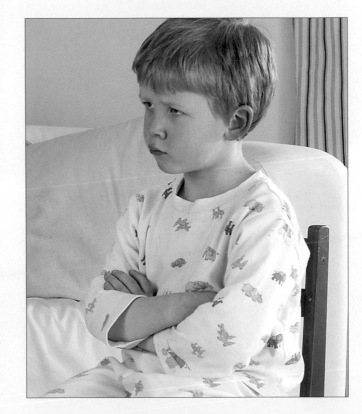

Top: As children's lives develop, people other than you will bring stimulus and interest. Your preschool child will benefit from these expanding horizons.

A young child is still likely to be unreasonable and grumpy, but uncontrollable tantrums should lessen as he or she becomes more able to communicate.

Food and the preschooler

Young children can be surprisingly sensible eaters. If you offer them lots of healthy foods, they will generally take enough for their needs and select a reasonably balanced diet. So even if your child is one of the many who turns his or her nose up at vegetables, you will probably find that a reliable liking for several types of fruit compensates for this.

Helping your child to develop a positive relationship with food is part of good parenting, but it isn't always easy, especially as your child starts to socialize more. Relatives and friends are bound to offer sweets, crisps and so on from time to time. Three to five year olds will probably be exposed to advertising for junk foods that is deliberately targeted at them. And they are likely to see other children eating these foods, which will naturally make them want to have some too.

The best way to cultivate your child's interest in good food is to involve him or her in choosing or preparing it. Even a trip to a supermarket can be fun.

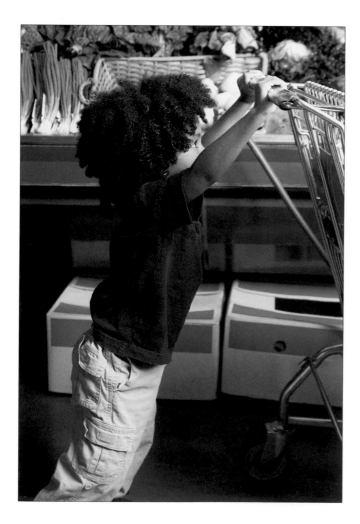

Children learn best by example, so to absorb the rudiments of table etiquette your child should share family mealtimes. Around the age of four, a child learns to handle a knife and fork well, but this is easier if they are special child-sized ones.

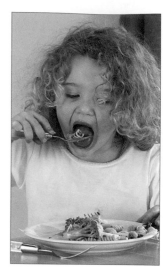

ESTABLISHING GOOD EATING HABITS

To help your child take a sensible and positive attitude to food, you need to set a good example yourself. If choosing and eating good nutritious food is the norm in your household, your children will naturally be inclined to adopt good eating habits. Explain that certain foods are good for you and others aren't, but don't give your child long lectures about healthy eating: he or she will switch off. Instead, get your child involved in choosing and preparing food to help develop an interest in it: let him or her pick out which fruit to buy when you are shopping and do some simple cooking together.

Avoid loading particular foods with emotional significance. People often give children sweets as rewards or bribes for good behaviour or to cheer them up when they are upset. It's better if your child views them just as another pleasant food. Equally, don't ban foods completely or you will make them seem even more desirable. An occasional trip to a fast-food restaurant won't ruin your child's palate.

Choose healthier snack foods: baked low-salt pretzels are better than flavoured crisps; chocolate, which quickly melts in the mouth, is better than boiled sweets, which linger. Have plenty of healthy snacks available: dried fruit,

IRON
Some preschool children don't get enough iron. The richest sources are red meat, but eggs, red kidney beans, canned fish, dried fruit and green leafy vegetables are also good. Serve foods rich in vitamin C at the same time to help the body absorb the iron.

BRAIN FOOD

Give your child two portions of fish a week, including one portion of oily fish such as salmon, mackerel, trout or tuna. Fish oils have been shown to help with concentration, social skills and behaviour.

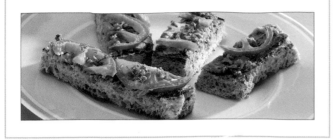

Milk and other dairy foods are still an important part of your child's diet: give three servings a day. A 200ml/$^{1}/_{3}$ pint glass of milk, a pot of yoghurt and a chunk of cheese provides your child with enough calcium.

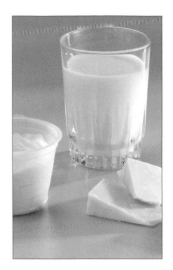

sticks of cheese, fresh fruit, mini-sandwiches, oatcakes, rice cakes and so on, and allow your child free access to these foods.

Give your child lots of water to drink as well as milk. If you want to give juice, dilute it well (one part juice to five parts water) and restrict it to mealtimes. Don't keep fizzy drinks (soda) or sweetened fruit drinks at home. If your child occasionally has these when out, try to make sure they are the ordinary versions rather than diet ones: the latter contain artificial sweeteners (such as aspartame), which are not recommended for young children.

Don't give your child ready-made convenience foods, which tend to be high in salt and made with inferior ingredients. You can make your own, much healthier versions of popular children's dishes: for example make chicken nuggets by dipping organic chicken pieces in whisked egg white then rolling them in breadcrumbs and baking in the oven; grill your own burgers, which are easily made from lean mince, wholemeal breadcrumbs, minced onions and herbs, bound together with egg. Roast thick-cut chips in the oven rather than fry them, and blot off the oil with kitchen paper, if you want to.

CHILDREN AND WEIGHT

Toddlers gradually slim down as they grow up, but you'll notice that your preschool child gets tubbier from time to time. This is because a child's body is designed to put on weight (puppy fat) just before a growth spurt. The energy stored in the fat will be burned off as it fuels the growing process. A small proportion of children put on weight without gaining height. This is the first step towards childhood obesity, an ever more acute problem in modern society. So if your child is overweight, you should address this, but follow these important guidelines.

Don't put a young child on a diet. It is better for a child to grow into the weight than to try to lose it.

Don't talk about losing weight. Don't comment on your child's body in a negative way.

Do increase physical activity. Do something active every day: get out to the park more often, play chasing games, go swimming, get your child a bike.

Do maintain healthy food habits, but still allow your child other treats from time to time.

Do give semi-skimmed milk rather than full-fat milk.

Do give small portions at mealtimes. Give your child another helping if he or she wants it, but never push extra food on your child or insist that everything is eaten.

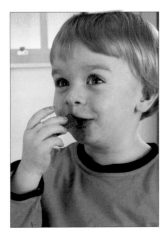
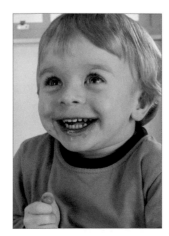

Banning sweet treats altogether is likely to be counterproductive – the occasional piece of chocolate will give huge enjoyment.

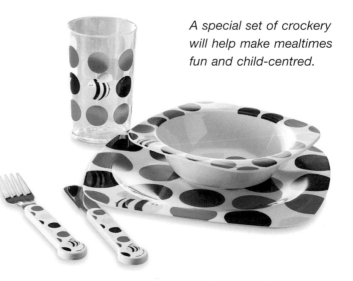

A special set of crockery will help make mealtimes fun and child-centred.

Sleep for preschool children

Many preschool children positively enjoy going to bed. Unlike toddlers, who don't like to be separated from their parents, older children can really appreciate the calm and routine of bedtime.

The need for sleep varies from child to child, but most preschool children need 11–13 hours' sleep a night. If your child doesn't get enough sleep, he or she is likely to be tired and irritable during the day. And your sleep will inevitably be affected, too. To encourage good sleeping habits, stick to a set bedtime and have a consistent bedtime routine. Help your child to wind down by avoiding rough play and noisy games and ruling out television, which can be physically and emotionally stimulating, for the hour before bedtime. Help your child to make a calm transition by giving a warning that bedtime is coming up. While young children probably need a five-minute warning followed by a one-minute

Reading a story together before bed is a wonderful way for your child to wind down and to enjoy being close to you at the end of the day.

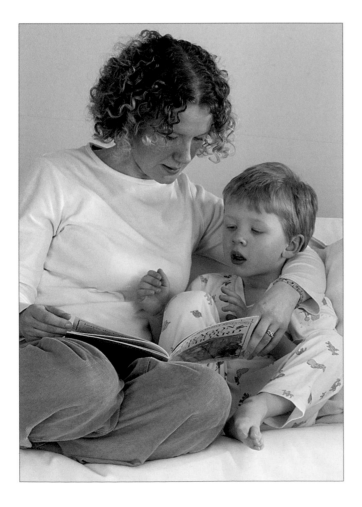

DAYTIME NAPS

Some children continue to have a daytime nap until they go to school, but most have stopped napping by the age of four. When your child first gives up a daytime nap, he or she is bound to get tired and irritable by the end of the day. You can help to manage this fatigue by ensuring that your child has regular meals and snacks and drinks lots of fluid. Balancing physical activities with quieter ones will also help. Some parents find that their preschool children are happy to go to bed for half an hour or so after lunch for some "quiet time" instead of a nap: this is a great habit to instil.

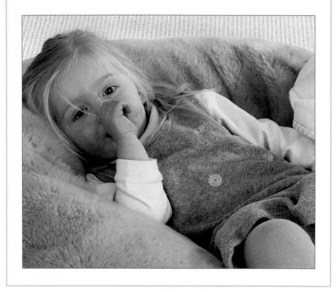

warning, older children benefit from longer warnings (15–30 minutes), and may want to choose a final activity before the bedtime routine starts. Give your child your undivided attention as he or she prepares for bed. Most children love their bedtime story and goodnight kiss. Bedtime is also a valuable opportunity for your child to tell you about the day or confide something that is worrying him or her.

Be clear that lights-out means sleep time, and don't let your child string out bedtime by asking for "one more story". Leave your child to drop off alone, but for reassurance say that you'll be back in five minutes to check if he or she is asleep. If the child is still awake when you go back, say you'll be back in another five minutes. Have a firm rule that once in bed, your child stays there and should call you if he or she needs anything. The exception is needing to go to the bathroom.

SLEEP PROBLEMS

Some sleep disturbances are a fact of childhood: a nationwide survey of American children found that about 70 per cent experienced one or more of the following sleep problems most weeks.

Nightmares. Children between three and five have vivid imaginations but don't yet understand where the boundary lies between the physical world and their own inner universe, so nightmares are common. They need swift comfort and reassurance after a bad dream. It's important to tell your child that dreams aren't real and can't hurt, but you may need to switch on the light so that you can prove that there are, say, no monsters in the room. A small number of children have regular nightmares, which may be triggered by stress, changes in their routine or upsetting events. Helping children to talk about how they are feeling is helpful, and comforters and nightlights provide extra reassurance.

Night terrors. Unlike nightmares, which happen late at night, night terrors tend to occur an hour or two after the child has gone to sleep. They can be scary to witness because the child's eyes are open but he or she appears to be terrified. Don't try to wake your child, but stay with him or her. The child will settle when the dream ends, and won't remember it the next day. Night terrors can be connected with lack of sleep, so making bedtime earlier may help. Factors such as stress and sleeping in a strange environment can also trigger them.

Sleepwalking. Sleepwalking is very common in children. They usually do it an hour or two after going to bed. Don't wake a child who is sleepwalking, but make sure he or

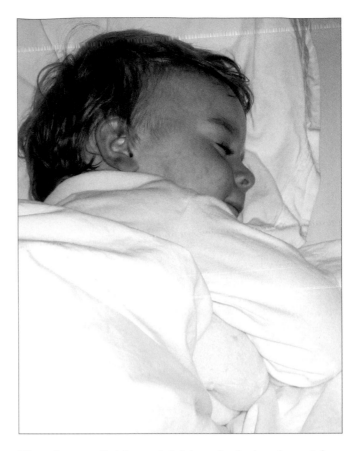

Sleep is essential for maintaining physical and mental health, so it is important to teach your child good sleeping habits from an early age.

Make sure your child has calmed down before you begin the bedtime routine. If he or she is involved in a game, give a warning that bath time is in five minutes.

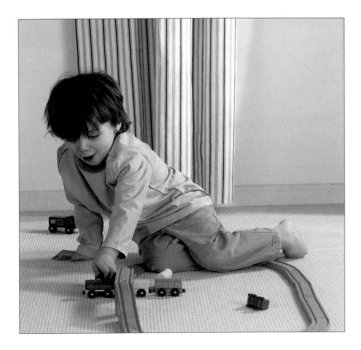

she cannot come to any harm. Sleepwalking is associated with lack of sleep.

Snoring. Most children snore from time to time, and around 10 per cent snore often. If your child snores regularly and loudly, and also seems to have difficulty breathing, he or she could have sleep apnoea. In this condition, the child momentarily stops breathing and starts suddenly with a gasp or snort. This stop-start breathing affects sleep, so your child may be cranky or tired during the day. If you think your child may have sleep apnoea, see your doctor for a referral to a sleep specialist.

YOUR CHILD'S BEDROOM

It will help your child to sleep well if he or she sees their bedroom as a pleasant place to be, so don't use it as a place to send them as punishment. A nicely decorated room that is kept reasonably tidy and clean is naturally appealing, and you can choose an attractive bedcover that your child will like – or you can let him or her choose it. Keep a selection of toys and books within reach of the bed, so that he or she can amuse himself when he wakes up. A light that he or she can switch on from the security of the bed can help a feeling of security. If he or she is scared of the dark or has nightmares, then try leaving a dim nightlight on. He or she may have a special soft toy or comfort object that you can suggest they sleep with.

Physical and mental development

Three year olds have mastered the basic physical skills: they can walk, run, jump and climb easily. But can still be clumsy and uncoordinated. Over the next year or two, their balance will improve to the extent that they can walk along a low wall without falling off it. They'll also learn to hop (some time around their fourth birthday), but skipping – a complicated movement – will take longer to master. They may learn to ride a bike if given lots of help.

The upper body gets much stronger and children learn to pull themselves up by their hands. If they are confident in the water, they may learn to swim. It's a good idea to get your child into the habit of having lots of physical activity at an early age, so get out to the park and play plenty of games, chase and so on.

Hand and finger control become more precise: by the age of four, children tend to grasp a pen between thumb and finger as adults do. This allows them to draw with much greater accuracy: a four year old can usually copy simple geometric shapes and colour inside the lines. Everyday tasks such as getting dressed, putting on shoes and washing the face and hands will be achieved more easily, though adult help is often needed. Some children are able to clean their own teeth at four or five, but still need supervision.

Developmental reviews (well-child visits) will check hearing, eyesight and progress, and give you an opportunity to discuss your child's daily life.

Many children learn to recognize numbers from quite a young age and may like to play simple number-recognition games such as dominoes.

WATCHING TELEVISION

Children over the age of three can benefit from watching some television: research by the American Academy of Pediatrics found that children who watched educational television actually did better in some maths and language tests. But too much television will stop them learning through more active play, so limit your child to an hour's viewing a day, of children's videos or educational programmes.

MENTAL PROGRESS

Preschool children gradually gain much better recall of recent events. Their sense of time is also developing, and their new ability to think about future events means that they can start to plan ahead.

Language develops rapidly now and most young children enjoy learning new words. Your conversations will get more interesting and you'll notice that your child starts to use adjectives and adverbs as well as nouns and verbs. He or she will enjoy all sorts of language play: made-up words, silly songs, jokes, rhymes and stories.

Your child can now express curiosity about the world in language, so prepare to be bombarded with questions. "Why?" is the familiar cry of the preschool child. Answer these questions as simply as you can, and keep your language at a level they can understand. Sometimes children ask why? to continue the conversation rather than because they want a specific answer. Encourage your child to frame a genuine query in a whole sentence.

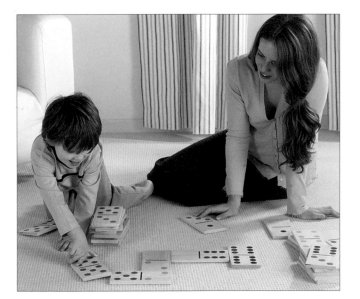

TEACHING NUMBERS AND LETTERS

You don't need to teach your preschool child to read or do sums, but it is helpful to get him or her familiar with letters and numbers. Show your child the letters that make up his or her name: stick magnetic letters or numbers on the fridge. Help your child learn about numbers by pointing out that he or she is playing with two teddies, but only one doll, for example; look at house and bus numbers when you are out and about.

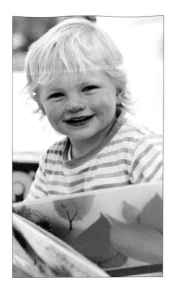

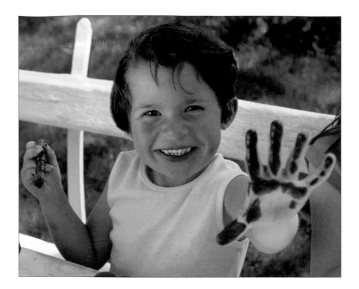

Left: If books are a part of a baby's life right from the early months, it is likely that your developing toddler will entertain himself or herself by looking at the pictures in books, as well as asking you to read the story.

Right: At first, children paint for the fun of it, then they give their art a label. Finally they draw something specific.

TOYS AND GAMES

Choose toys with long-lasting appeal, which can be used in different ways as your child gets older. Good toys for this age group include dolls, extendable railway sets, small construction blocks, balls, musical instruments and non-toxic felt-tip pens. Avoid buying toy guns: a young boy will almost certainly make his own make-believe weapons using his fingers or sticks, but research shows that having toy guns encourages aggressive play. Preschool children enjoy make-believe. They want to play at being other people, rather than just imitating their parents' actions, as toddlers do. Expect to see your mannerisms exaggerated in games of mummies and daddies and to see some rather sexist divisions of labour.

Three and four year olds can get a lot out of playing board games or simple card games, such as "pairs", in which they have to turn over matching picture cards. These games naturally involve turn-taking, and they also are a good way to introduce the concept of winning and losing. But losing is hard for most children, so it is good to let them win most of the time.

ENJOYING BOOKS AND MUSIC

Your child will get a lot out of story books: look out for books with detailed illustrations that offer more scope for discussion. It's also worth getting a couple of illustrated children's reference books: you are unlikely to be able to answer all the questions that your child has about the world, and it is good for children to see that books offer exciting information they want to know about.

Have fun with music: there's evidence to suggest that active music-making can help with language and mathematical ability, concentration and memory. Sing together (songs that involve movement are particularly good), get your child a musical instrument such as a keyboard, toy piano or xylophone, dance together (a child will love to stand on your feet and hold your hands while you dance), and look for a dance or creative movement class for under-fives in your area. Play recordings at home and seek out live music you can enjoy for short periods.

Your child is now old enough to do some simple cooking, which offers real-life practice in weighing, measuring and pouring.

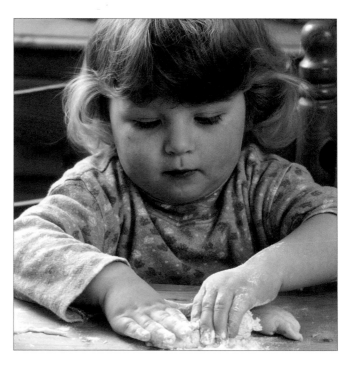

HOW CHILDREN DRAW PEOPLE
Children's representations of the human figure all follow the same progressive pattern. At first, children will draw a circle for the head with two vertical lines representing legs. They may add dots for eyes and marks for the mouth and nose. By four, a torso is usually present and the figure may have arms. By five, the figure has a trunk, arms have hands, legs have feet, and there may be clothing on the body.

Yoga for children

Yoga is a beautiful discipline that involves using the body in a completely different way to other forms of exercise. Children don't have the focus to practise it as adults do: you can't expect a preschooler to sit quietly for long. But they will get a lot out of a short yoga session that focuses on having fun.

BENEFITS OF YOGA

Children are naturally supple, but they start to stiffen up once they go to school and spend most of the day sitting, then spend lots of time watching television or playing computer games. Yoga helps them to stretch their bodies and maintain flexibility, good posture and muscle strength. It teaches good balance, coordination and natural awareness of the body, which can reduce clumsiness. It is non-competitive but can be challenging, so it can increase children's physical confidence.

Lots of the poses are based on animal movements or other elements of nature. Imagining themselves as different creatures, trees or mountains can help children to become more aware of their environment and more sensitive to it.

Yoga works on the mind as well as the body. It induces a feeling of natural calm and relaxation, and may help your child to sleep better. It also builds the mental focus of children, including those who are hyperactive. It teaches that being quiet can be enjoyable. There are lots

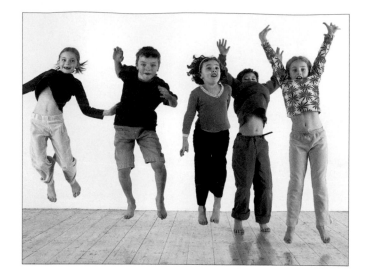

A good yoga class will offer an outlet for youthful exuberance and help children to channel their natural energy in a positive way.

of health benefits, too: yoga encourages good breathing (it may be helpful for those children who have asthma or get chesty), it also helps the digestion and boosts the immune system.

YOGA AT HOME

You don't have to be an expert to teach your child simple yoga poses. Find a quiet area of the home (or go outside), clear away clutter, which can be distracting, and make sure you are both able to stretch out safely. Wear comfortable clothing that doesn't restrict your movements, and have bare feet.

Do a quick warm-up by running on the spot or doing some star jumps to help your child release excess energy. Then try some of these poses: keep the atmosphere playful and move quite quickly from one posture to the next to keep your child interested. Getting your child to make noises (such as barking like a dog) or to imagine what each pose is based on will help him or her to maintain the poses for longer. Try to end the session with a few moments' rest.

CHILDREN'S YOGA CLASSES

A good yoga teacher for children will use the classic postures as the basis for games or to create a magical story: children may swim like fishes or roar like lions. Look for an atmosphere that is creative and dynamic. Some classes take children from the age of two, but most are for the over-threes.

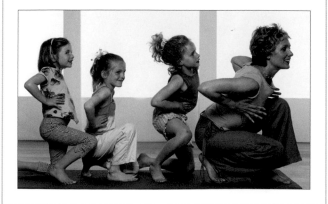

CAUTION

Don't get children doing headstands or shoulderstands – their neck muscles are not strong enough. Never push a child into a posture, or you could cause damage.

Cat stretch

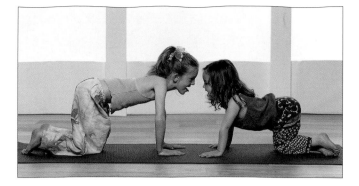

Go on to all fours, on your hands and knees; you are going to be cat who has just woken up. Stretch like a cat – let your head drop down and arch your back and stre-e-e-tch. Now bring your head up, let your back drop down and miaow, miaow, miaow. Do both again. Walk around the room being cats.

Dog pose

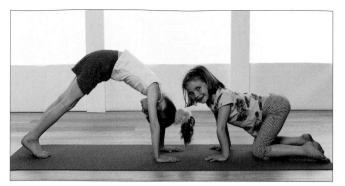

Get on to your hands and knees. Then go on to your toes and straighten your legs: you are a dog stretching after a sleep. Push your hands and your toes into the floor and stre-e-e-tch. Now imagine you see a tiny mouse under your nose: bark to shoo it away. Thank goodness, you can stretch again. Oh-oh, here comes the mouse again...

Roar like a lion

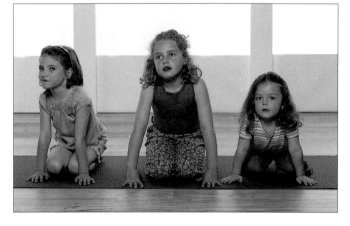

1 Kneel on the floor with your legs together, then sit back, with your hands on the floor in front of you.

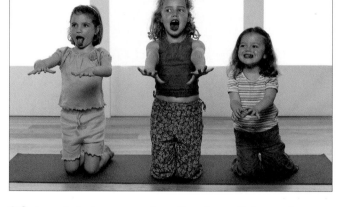

2 Get ready to be a scary lion. Kneel up, stick your tongue out and roar... "Raaaah!" Hold out those sharp claws.

Bridge

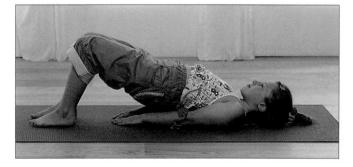

Lie on your back with your arms by your sides. Now bend your knees and bring your heels up to your bottom. Keep your feet and knees apart. Lift up your bottom and turn your body into a bridge: you've got to be really strong so that all the people can walk over you. Keep your bottom up: let the ships sail underneath you. Lower your bridge and repeat a couple more times.

Give yourself a cuddle

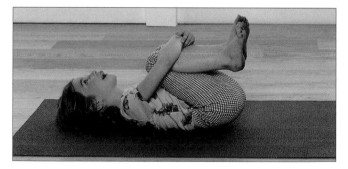

Lie on your back, bend your knees so that you can put your feet flat on the floor. Now bring up your knees so you can hug them. Give them a squeeze – bring them right to your chest: give yourself a lovely cuddle, mmmmmmm. Now try rocking from side to side, like you are a little turtle on its back: ooh this is comfy. Now stretch out your legs again and sl-ee-eeee-p.

Encouraging good behaviour

Small children don't have any real sense of what is right and what is wrong. But they do have a desire to please their parents or carers and they understand that older people have authority over them. You can channel your child's instinct to please you into good behaviour in the following ways.

Set a good example. Children love to imitate, and they naturally think that what you do is right. So you must set an example of good behaviour yourself: if you want your child to speak politely to others, you must do so too; if you don't want your child to shout or hit out at others, don't shout at or hit your child.

Encourage a level of responsibility. Give your child opportunities to help you: wiping up the drink he or she has spilled, fetching your bag when you are going out.

Acknowledge good behaviour. Show that you are pleased when your child is doing things that you approve of, such as giving another child some of his or her apple slices, or playing nicely with toys.

Disapprove of bad behaviour. When your child does something you dislike, say so. Keep it simple: "You kicked Ellie. Kicking is wrong because it hurts people." Talk about the behaviour as being wrong, rather than the child being "naughty" or "bad". Don't unintentionally "reward" bad behaviour by giving your child extra attention because of it.

BEHAVIOUR AND DIET
Lots of parents see a link between certain foods and their child's behaviour. Fizzy drinks (soda), processed foods and lots of sugar can all have a negative impact, while regular meals and healthy snacks help to regulate a child's blood sugar levels and moods. Fish oils have also been shown to have a beneficial effect on behaviour: a children's fish-oil supplement may be worth considering.

Be fair. Give your child the opportunity to learn what is unacceptable. A small child may be confused if you tell him or her off for, say, drawing on the walls when in the child's eyes it is no different from the perfectly permissible business of scribbling on an old newspaper. What is more, small children naturally believe that the naughtiness of a given action is related to the enormity of the consequences, rather than to the intention to do harm. So you need to make a distinction between deliberate acts (such as hitting others) and accidental ones (such as knocking over a vase). It will take time for this to sink in, so be patient, forgiving, consistent and persistent.

Stay in control. If you get angry, or shout at or smack your child, you have lost control. Your child may do what

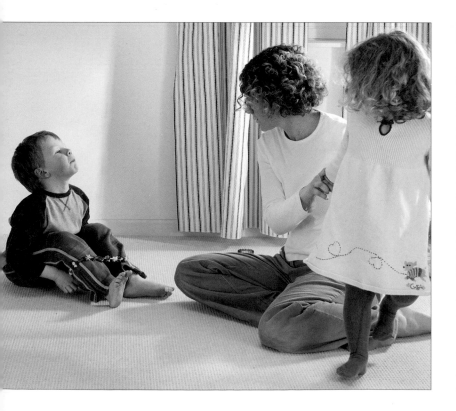

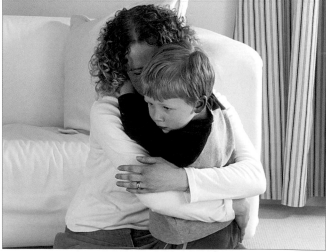

If there has been a dispute between two children, make sure that after you have mediated and reprimanded there is forgiveness. Make space and time for apologies and making up. Don't stay angry for too long on principle. Once you have made your point let everyone recover from it and move on.

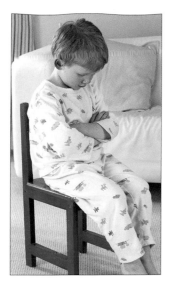

Time out is a great technique to help your child learn that their negative behaviour will have negative consequences. It isn't a punishment so much as a chance for your child to calm down and reflect on his or her actions.

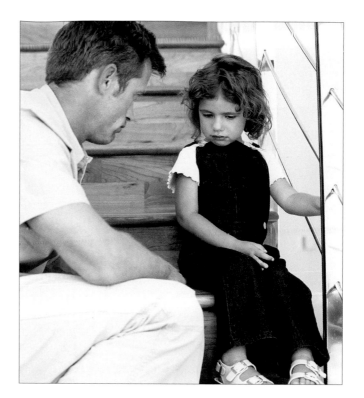

If you need to reprimand your child, squat down so that you are at the child's level. Say the behaviour is wrong in a calm but firm voice. Don't shout from on high.

you say from fear but this won't help him or her to learn how to behave well. If you think you are going to lose your temper, tell your child that you are getting angry and are leaving the room to calm down. And if you do lose it (as almost all parents do at some time), it's best to acknowledge the fact and apologize.

FEELING THE CONSEQUENCES

A good way to help preschool children develop better behaviour is to let them feel the consequences of their actions. If your child refuses to eat dinner, for example, you could try going out and not taking snacks with you. Once a child experiences the consequence of refusing food – being hungry – he or she may be more inclined to eat dinner next time.

The consequence has to be linked to the behaviour, and must be proportionate to it. So, you might let your child go out without food, but you won't keep him or her

out for hours. Keep your attitude calm and sympathetic – "What a shame you are hungry, that's probably because you didn't eat your dinner" will drive the message home.

THE TIME-OUT METHOD

If your child is doing something that he or she knows is wrong, then the time-out method can be very helpful. It involves putting the child in a safe place until he or she is ready to behave reasonably. To make it work, you have to observe all the steps, in the order given here. In particular, don't miss out the warning stage.

1 Tell your child not to do something: "Peter, stop kicking the table." If the behaviour continues, say, "Peter, I told you to stop kicking the table. You either stop now or go for some time out."

2 If the child does it again, remove him or her to your safe place: this could be a room with a door you can shut, the bottom stair or a quiet corner of the house. Tell the child he or she is to sit there until ready to behave nicely. Alternatively, tell your child to sit there for a set period – one minute for each year of age is a good formula: a four-year-old should stay for four minutes, and so on.

3 When your child comes out or time is up, ask him or her to say sorry. If the child does this, have a hug and make up. If the child refuses, put him or her back into the time-out spot and repeat until you get an apology.

5 Some children run out of the safe place immediately. Simply lead your child back again quietly and calmly, as often as it takes. Don't lose your cool.

LYING AND STEALING

Telling lies is very common in the over-threes: it is a sign of their growing imaginations and a normal developmental stage. Young children make up lots of fantastic stories because they have difficulty distinguishing between fact and fiction. They may also lie to get themselves out of trouble. It will help your child to be honest if you are understanding about naughtiness and don't overreact to misdemeanours or accidents.

Similarly, you may find that your child squirrels away things that don't belong to him or her. Young children have only a vague idea about possessions, so your child doesn't understand why this is wrong. Calmly explaining that we don't take things from other people because it makes them sad will help. In older children, stealing can sometimes be a sign that the child feels he or she is lacking attention or love.

Sociability in the wider world

Children gradually develop empathy from the age of about three: they realize that other people not only have feelings but may react or feel differently than they would do themselves in the same situations. Once they have made this intellectual leap, they are able to make proper friendships and their social skills improve. With your help, your child will start to show behaviour that is more cooperative and thoughtful.

ENCOURAGING FRIENDSHIPS

Friends will become increasingly important to your child from now on. Going to nursery or playgroup, or having regular playtimes with other children, will give your child lots of opportunities to interact with other children.

Teach your child to take turns and not to snatch things from another child. If small children are playing a game that involves turn-taking, an adult should supervise.

Your child needs to be able to voice his or her needs honestly. Children with good language skills naturally find it easier to manage in group situations, so set aside time each day to talk to your child without interruptions. Encourage a shy child to speak loudly and clearly. When with other children, try to get him or her to come up with solutions for conflict. Say something like, "You and Mike both want the toy and you are getting cross. How can we make both you and Mike happy?" Suggest taking turns, playing together, and other possible solutions if your child isn't able to come up with any.

Teach your child to stand up for himself or herself when necessary. Young children need to know that they can say "No" to another child or refuse to give up a toy if someone else tries to grab it. Practise ways of doing this in a reasonable way. But don't let your child think he or she has to do this all alone: children need to know that they can ask an adult for help. Help your child feel secure in a new situation, such as preschool nursery, by introducing him or her to it gradually and make sure he or she knows which adult is in charge in group situations.

Encourage empathy – helping children to recognize other people's feelings spurs them to be kind and cooperative. So say, "If you take Joey's tractor, he'll be sad." But alongside this encouragement to behave well, let your child know that you understand that doing things for other people can be difficult.

BOOSTING SELF-ESTEEM

Children who feel good about themselves naturally do well in group situations and will also cope better with the challenges of school. Here are some ways to boost self-esteem in your child.

- Talk to your child about what is special about him or her.
- Point out things that your child is good at.
- Don't tease your child about things he or she finds difficult; be sympathetic.
- Encourage your child to talk about his or her emotions.
- Make sure your child knows that he or she is loved even when behaving badly: it is the behaviour that you don't like, not the child.
- Show your child that his or her opinions are important by listening and acknowledging what he or she says (even if you don't do what the child wants).
- Give your child some sense of mastery over a situation by letting him or her make simple choices between two or three equally satisfactory options.

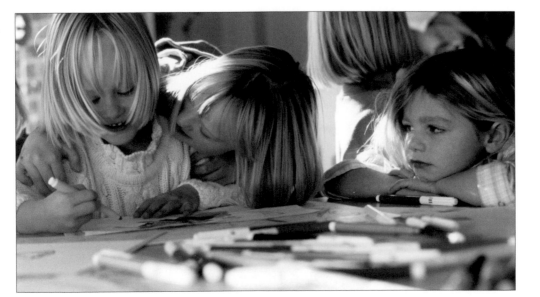

If you feel your child is struggling to integrate at nursery, talk to him or her about ways to start an interaction with someone else: try telling a story about another child who wants to join in a game, and get your child to suggest some strategies.

CHOOSING A NURSERY

Some group care can be beneficial for children over the age of three because it gives them the opportunity to develop good social skills before they go to school. It also sets up a positive pattern for learning. An American study that followed children through their early school years found that those who received high-quality nursery care did better in language and maths. They also tended to have better concentration, were more sociable and demonstrated less problem behaviour. If you are choosing a nursery for your child, look for one where:

- the atmosphere is friendly and happy
- the nursery is clean and well-organized
- the children seem to be enjoying their activities
- the children seem happy to make requests from staff
- the staff speak warmly about and to their charges
- the majority of staff are trained
- the facilities and activities on offer suit your child's personality – for example, for a very active child, look for a nursery with a soft room and outdoor play area.

STARTING NURSERY

If your child has never been to nursery before, it is bound to feel strange at first. It will help your child to cope if he or she is already used to being in groups of children (such as parent-and-toddler groups).

Attend a trial session so that your child can meet the staff and learn where everything is while you are there. Stay in the background as much as possible. If your child seems to be settling happily, then tell him or her you are going out (to visit the shops) and will be back soon. Say goodbye calmly and confidently – it won't help your child cope if he or she can see that you are worried about leaving, and sneaking off without saying you are going will

Learning to manage in a group situation is an essential life skill. Going to preschool can give your child valuable experience of this before he or she goes to school.

MALE ROLE MODELS

Most children are cared for by their mothers, and nursery workers and preschool teachers are also predominantly female. It's important that children spend time playing with their fathers, and that those whose fathers are absent most or all of the time develop strong relationships with other trustworthy male relatives or family friends. This is particularly important for boys. It's also very good for young boys if their fathers read to them and, later on, take an interest in their schoolwork.

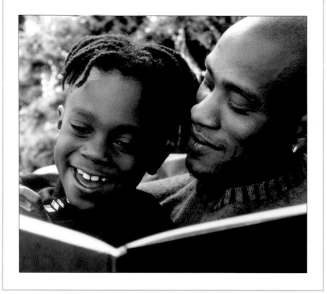

shake your child's confidence. Make a judgment on how long to stay away: err on the side of caution the first time.

Some children need a few trial sessions: gradually increase the length of time you leave the nursery. If your child cries when you leave, call to check whether he or she has settled soon afterwards (most children do). It can be helpful to follow the same "goodbye" and "hello" ritual each day to ease the stress of the transition, and many children like to keep a favourite toy with them.

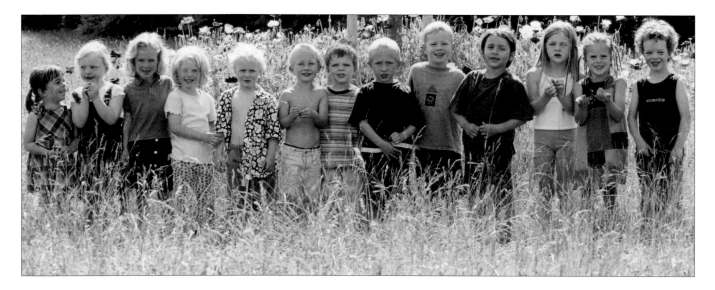

Health and safety

“ Children need to feel loved and secure in order to develop good mental health, which also contributes to physical well-being. ”

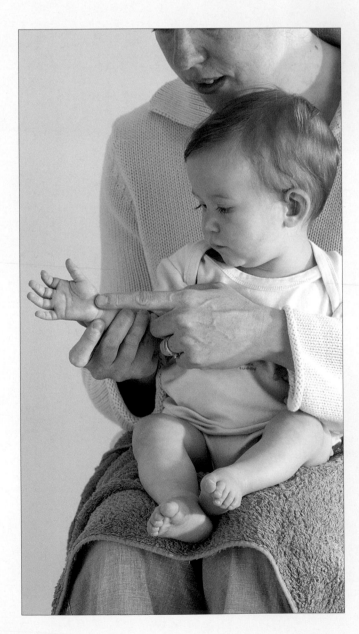

A healthy lifestyle will go a long way towards making your child's immune system strong, so that he or she can fight off bugs and recover from minor ailments quickly.

Give your child a healthy balanced diet of home-cooked food. Using fresh, locally produced, organic produce will minimize the amount of pesticides your child is exposed to and will help to ensure he or she gets as many nutrients as possible. Fresh garlic in the diet is helpful: it has natural antibiotic properties. Encourage your child to drink lots of water. Proper hydration is essential for general well-being, and may help reduce the risk of disease. Filter tap water before giving it to your child if you can.

It's important to facilitate good sleeping habits. Children need a lot more sleep than adults: up to 16 hours for newborns, and around 12 hours for three-year-olds. And make exercise part of your child's daily life. Most children spend about 90 per cent of their time indoors, so some physical activity outdoors will build muscle strength and get them

Natural remedies such as aromatherapy oils can relieve common symptoms, but check that your child won't react to them by doing a patch test before use.

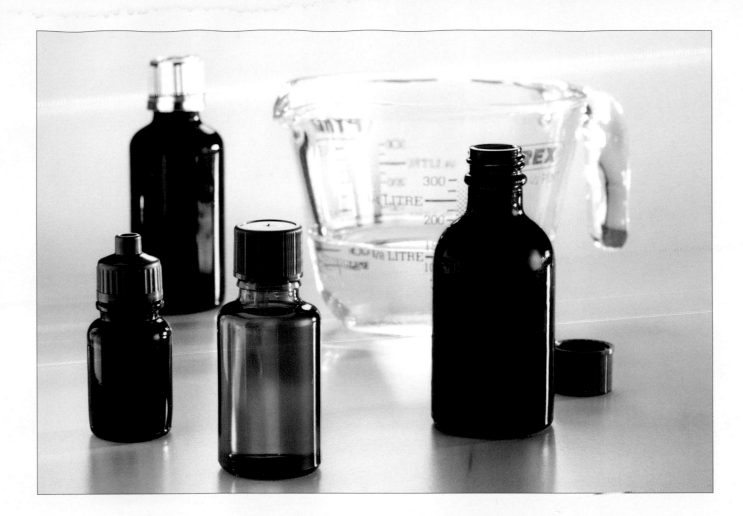

breathing fresh air. Babies benefit from being taken out every day and from spending time on the floor, where they can move their arms and legs freely.

Make your home as healthy an environment as possible, by reducing your use of chemical-laden household products and taking basic safety precautions. Avoid unnecessary risks. Observe basic hygiene when preparing your child's food to prevent stomach upsets, and keep your child away from people with infectious diseases.

Finally, give your child lots of unreserved love and affection. It's known that babies need plenty of physical contact in order to thrive; children, too, need to feel loved, valued and secure in order to develop good mental health, which also contributes to physical well-being.

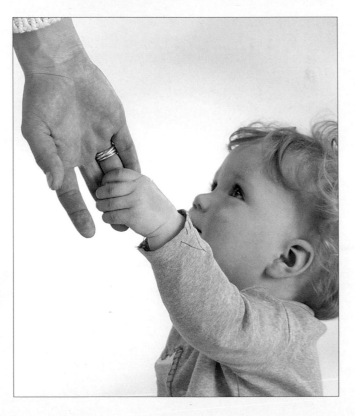

Top: Reducing the amount of noxious chemicals you use in the home is an important aspect of healthy living. For a natural air freshener, try aromatherapy oils.

All parents want to do the best for their children, and an abundance of love and affection lays the foundation for good mental health.

health and safety

Immunization and supplements

The subject of immunization causes parents a lot of anxiety, but in a sense there is nothing unnatural about it: what you are doing is introducing a small dose of a disease into the body so that the immune system can develop antibodies to it. This is exactly what the body does when it encounters a disease "accidentally", except that with vaccination the body does not go through the dangers and unpleasantness of illness.

There is no doubt that we all have benefited from a widespread vaccination programme: smallpox has been eradicated worldwide, and diseases such as polio and diphtheria are now largely unknown in developed countries. However, there is much debate about the wisdom of vaccinating very young children. Some natural practitioners say that the standard practice of immunizing babies against several diseases at once overloads their immature immune systems and can lead to an increased risk of problems such as asthma, eczema and allergy later on. And parents worry about the possibility of side effects. Controversy over the MMR jab, which was linked to autism in one British study, caused many parents to decide not to give it to their children. This study has been widely discredited and intensive research has not found a link. Generally speaking, the risk of serious side effects from a vaccine is much smaller than the risk from diseases such as measles.

Every parent has to make an individual decision about what is right for a child. There are four options:

Following the standard vaccination programme. This is what the vast majority of doctors recommend.

Delaying vaccinations. Some people prefer to give vaccinations when the child is older, to give the immune system a chance to strengthen. This may make you feel more comfortable, especially if there is a family history

of allergy or allergy-related illnesses. However, your child will obviously not be protected in the meantime.

Having selected vaccinations. Some parents prefer to avoid giving children all-in-one shots, and choose not to vaccinate against certain diseases. It is worth bearing in mind that single-vaccine injections may not have been tested as rigorously as the standard injections.

Not vaccinating. If you feel strongly that vaccination is not right for your child, then you may decide not to do it

VACCINATION AFTER-EFFECTS

Your child may experience some minor side effects after a vaccination: fever, feeling irritable, and redness and soreness in the injection site are common. Call your doctor if his or her temperature goes above 39°C/102°F. Some children have an allergic reaction after the immunization; for this reason, you will asked to wait in the doctor's surgery for a short period after the injection has been given.

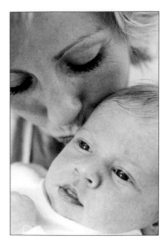

Vaccination jabs are usually given in the thigh. Some children barely notice them; others get upset but can usually be quickly soothed.

Giving children a specially developed multi-vitamin supplement will ensure that they receive the right amount of vitamins and minerals in their diet.

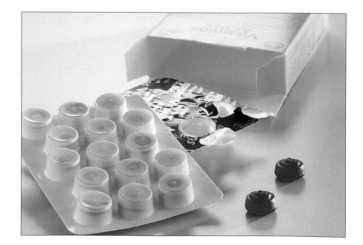

THE IMMUNIZATION PROGRAMME (UK)

2 months	One shot for diphtheria, tetanus, pertussis (whooping cough), haemophilus influenza B (HIB), polio One shot for meningitis C	4 months	Diphtheria, tetanus, pertussis (2/5) HIB (2/4) Polio (2/4) PCV7 (2/4)
3 months	One shot for diphtheria, tetanus, pertussis, HIB One shot for meningitis C	6 months	Diphtheria, tetanus, pertussis (3/5) HIB (3/4) PCV7 (3/4)
4 months	One shot for diphtheria, tetanus, pertussis, HIB, polio One shot for meningitis C	12 months	Hepatitis B (3/3) Varicella (chickenpox) MMR (1/2)
13 months	Measles, mumps and rubella (MMR)	6–23 months	Influenza (annual shot)
3–5 years	One shot for diphtheria, tetanus, pertussis, HIB One shot for MMR	15–18 months	HIB (4/4) Polio (3/4) PCV7 (4/4) Diphtheria, tetanus, pertussis (4/5)

THE IMMUNIZATION PROGRAMME (US)

Birth–2 months	Hepatitis B (1/3)	2 years +	Hepatitis A, for specific groups only (1/2)
2 months	Diphtheria, tetanus, pertussis (1/5) HIB (1/4) Polio (1/4) Hepatitis B (2/3) Pneumococcal conjugate (PCV7) (1/4)	2 1/2 years +	Hepatitis A, for specific groups only (2/2)
		2–5 years	Pneumococcal polysaccharide (PPV23), high risk only (1/2)
		4–6 years	Diphtheria, tetanus, pertussis (5/5) Polio (4/4) MMR (2/2)

at all. Ensuring your child is as healthy as possible is vital: a child with a robust immune system is likely to react to infection less severely. Seek advice from a naturopath, nutritional therapist or homeopath on ways to help support your child's immune system.

NUTRITIONAL SUPPLEMENTS FOR CHILDREN

Many nutritionists maintain that you can get all the nutrients you need from a good mixed diet. However, the mineral and vitamin content of fresh produce has dropped in recent years as the soil in which food is grown has become depleted. Giving children a daily multimineral, multivitamin supplement helps to ensure that they get enough health-giving trace elements, such as zinc.

Minerals work in combination inside the body, so it is not a good idea to give single mineral supplements without professional advice: giving a dose of one mineral could lead to a deficiency in another. Giving high doses of certain vitamins can also be dangerous. If you think that your child needs a particular nutrient, it is best to seek advice from a qualified nutritional therapist or your doctor.

Probiotics work to replenish levels of good bacteria in the gut, which help with digestion. They can be very useful if your child has had a stomach upset or been on

A liquid vitamin formulation, which is gentle on the stomach and suitable for children, can be bought from health food stores; babies can be given vitamin drops.

antibiotics. Fish oils (omega-3), or a vegetarian equivalent such as flaxseed, can be beneficial if your child will not eat oily fish. A deficiency in omega-3 oils may contribute to behavioural problems (including hyperactivity) and conditions such as eczema and asthma.

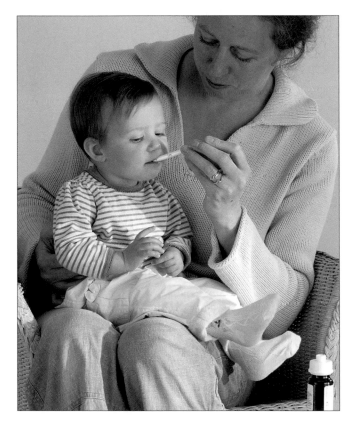

Natural medication

There's no doubt that modern medicine can be useful when your child is very ill. But it is wise to refrain from giving medication when it is not strictly necessary. Some medicines – such as cough mixtures – interrupt the workings of the immune system. Others, such as antibiotics, tend to be overused to the extent that they can be rendered impotent.

Natural remedies and common-sense measures can be just as good as conventional medicines in soothing certain symptoms and encouraging healing. And complementary therapies can encourage the body's natural ability to mend itself. Parents often feel more comfortable using natural methods to treat their children because they tend to have a gentler action than conventional medicines. But it is essential to take a balanced view. For example, not all natural remedies are gentle: some are toxic if taken in large quantities or are not advisable for babies or young children. And if your child is seriously ill, natural remedies are unlikely to help and urgent medical attention should always be sought.

GIVING MEDICATION

If possible, find a doctor who is open-minded and try to build a good and respectful relationship so that you can discuss alternative methods. If you know that your doctor generally agrees with a cautious approach to medication, you will also feel more confident about taking advice if he or she urges conventional treatment.

When your child is poorly they will probably become more clingy. If this helps comfort them it is probably the best way you can help them become well, especially if it helps them sleep – nature's best cure.

Always ask how a medicine works if you are going to give it to your child. You should know why you are giving it. Ask whether there are any side effects, so you can be on the lookout for them. If your child is already on medication – or is taking natural remedies – always mention it to the doctor. Check that the medicine is really necessary in your child's case. Sometimes a doctor may prescribe medication because that is what most parents expect, not because he or she feels it is essential treatment. Ask whether alternative medicines or approaches could work. Your doctor may be happy for you to delay giving antibiotics, say, for 24 hours to see if your child's condition improves on its own.

When you do give medication, don't forget to give every dose on time. Set an alarm to remind you, and keep a record of every dose you give. Don't stop the medication if your child starts to feel better. Antibiotics, for example, need to be taken for a set number of days in order to kill the bacteria and prevent infection recurring. On the other hand, sometimes the recommended course is longer than necessary, to allow for a margin of error: check with your doctor.

HIGH TEMPERATURE

The conventional response to a temperature is to give paracetamol (acetaminophen) to bring it down again. It is worth considering whether this is necessary, and whether simple natural measures may be sufficient. Fever is part of the body's natural response to infection. It helps to increase the number of disease-fighting white blood cells in the bloodstream, and boosts the level of the antiviral substance interferon. Once the immune system has beaten the infection, the temperature will return to normal.

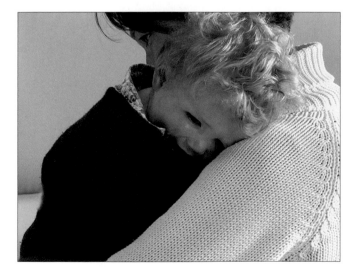

CAUTION
A very high temperature in a child can cause a fit (febrile convulsion). In the event of a seizure, lay your child on one side and remove anything in his or her

*Poorly children need lots of fluids to prevent dehydration.
A refreshing squeeze of lemon adds a little natural antiseptic to*

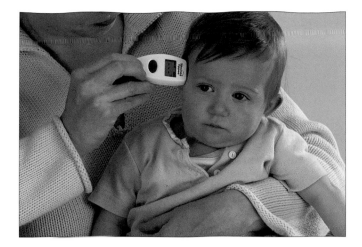

When your child has a fever there are ways you can bring it down without using drugs. Keep a close eye on them, though, and check their temperature frequently.

Your child needs a strong immune system in order to cope with all the bugs he or she comes across in daily life. One study found that the more fevers children had in the first year of life, the less likely they were to develop allergies later on. So it may be unwise to give medicines that, in the long term, may interfere with this natural mechanism for dealing with disease.

WHEN TO CALL A DOCTOR
Seek medical advice if a baby under three months has a fever, or if a child has a fever that is over 39°C/102°F, lasts

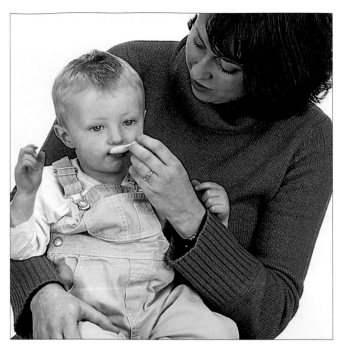

Older babies and children may prefer to take medicine from a spoon rather than a syringe; use a proper measuring spoon to be sure of giving the correct dose.

for longer than 24 hours or seems to be steadily increasing. If you do decide to give medication, children's paracetamol (acetaminophen), suitable for babies over two months, is milder than children's ibuprofen. Never give a child aspirin, which is linked with the rare and potentially fatal disease Reye's syndrome.

MANAGING FEVER NATURALLY
A fever can be dangerous if it gets very high and a raised temperature can also be uncomfortable. Follow these steps to help to lower a fever naturally.

1 Remove your child's clothing. Turn down any heating and ventilate the room to cool it.

2 Sponge your child down using tepid water; don't use cold water, as this will cause the blood vessels to contract, and so raise the core temperature of the body. Leave the water to evaporate rather than drying with a towel.

3 Dress your child in minimum clothing and, if he or she is in bed, cover with a sheet or light blanket. Give lots of fluid: frequent breastfeeds or extra drinks of cooled, boiled water for a baby; lots of cool drinks for older children. Encourage your child to sip drinks, as gulping could induce vomiting.

4 Check your child's temperature in half an hour, and then every hour or two.

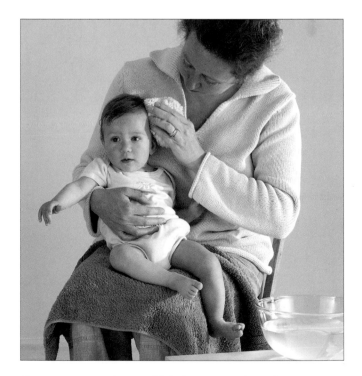

If you are sponging a child down to reduce fever, try adding 2 drops of lavender or chamomile essential oil mixed with 20ml/4 tsp full-fat milk to the water: these oils can help to reduce fever and encourage sleep.

Complementary therapies for children

Two types of treatment constitute complementary medicine. On the one hand, there are natural remedies that can be used to target particular ailments or symptoms, such as herbal teas and tinctures, essential oils, certain homeopathic pills and herbal creams. On the other hand, there are therapies such as acupuncture, osteopathy and homeopathy.

Natural therapies are holistic – they treat the body as a whole rather than targeting specific parts or symptoms. The body is seen as an organic and complex system in which an ailment may be caused by an imbalance in many parts; conversely many of the body's systems may need to be brought to bear to cure a specific hurt or sickness. For this reason, two children who seem to have the same symptoms may be given different treatments or remedies by the same complementary health practitioner.

There is often an assumption that natural remedies and therapies are always gentle and safe. But any treatment that is effective can be harmful if used incorrectly. Children can be more vulnerable to any side effects than adults, because their bodies are small and still developing. So it is essential to use complementary therapies and natural remedies wisely. Always check unusual symptoms with a doctor first.

USING COMPLEMENTARY THERAPIES SAFELY

When seeking treatment for your child, choose a complementary therapist who is qualified and trained. If possible, find one who specializes in treating children. Ask your doctor or other parents for a recommendation (but don't rely solely on someone else's opinion).

Where possible, pick a practitioner with several years' experience and make sure the therapist you choose is registered with the relevant professional association and that he or she is insured. Follow your instincts. If you do

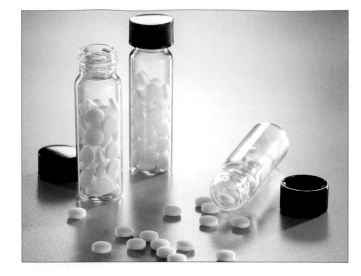

Always check that any natural remedy you buy over the counter is safe for children. If in doubt, or if your child has a chronic condition or severe symptoms, consult the relevant therapist. Check that the dosage is correct for your child.

not feel comfortable with a particular therapist, don't let him or her treat your child. Beware of anyone promising miraculous results.

Tell your doctor about any natural therapies your child is having: some remedies can interfere with conventional medication. Likewise, always tell a complementary therapist about any medication your child is taking. Do not stop your child's medication because he or she is having complementary treatment.

HOMEOPATHY

Homeopathic medicine uses very gentle remedies derived from natural ingredients (plants, minerals and animal substances such as bee venom). The remedies have been

AROMATHERAPY FOR CHILDREN

Age	Suitable oils	Recommended dosage
0–3 months	Do not use essential oils	
3–6 months	Lavender and Roman chamomile	1 drop per 10ml/2 tsp carrier oil or full-fat milk, or use in a vaporizer
6–12 months	Lavender, Roman chamomile, mandarin, neroli, rose	1 drop per 10ml/2 tsp carrier oil or full-fat milk, or use in a vaporizer
12 months–3 years	Lavender, chamomile, tea tree, mandarin, neroli, orange, rose, rosewood	2 drops per 10ml/2 tsp carrier oil or full-fat milk, or use in a vaporizer

diluted many times over, so that only a minuscule part of the active ingredient remains. However, homeopaths say this is enough to stimulate the immune system and encourage the body's natural ability to heal itself. Homeopathy can be used for a wide range of childhood complaints, including teething, sleeplessness, digestive complaints, coughs and colds. Many doctors refer patients to homeopaths, and some are trained in homeopathy in addition to conventional medicine.

Homeopathic remedies are available from health food stores and pharmacists, so home treatment is possible, but homeopathic remedies are prescribed not just on the basis of the symptoms but also according to personality, habits, build and so on. For this reason, it is usually better to consult a qualified homeopath, who can prescribe the correct constitutional remedy for your child.

A homeopath can also advise you on dosage. The paradox at the heart of homeopathy is that the more diluted the remedy the more powerful its effects: a remedy marked 200c is more dilute than one marked 6c. As a general rule, you should stick to remedies of 6c and 30c when treating at home. These are usually given three to six times a day, depending on the severity of the symptoms. Give 30c for no more than three days, 6c for up to a week, but stop when symptoms improve. Give one remedy at a time.

AROMATHERAPY

Essential oils, distilled or pressed from the flowers, leaves, bark or other parts of plants, have therapeutic properties, and can be helpful for skin problems, anxiety and sleeplessness. But they are highly concentrated so only a few are suitable for children. The best way to use

Natural and conventional approaches to health are not mutually exclusive and are often used side by side.

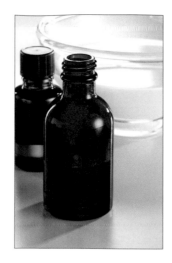

Essential oils should never be applied neat to a child's delicate skin. Always dilute them in either full-fat milk or in a suitable carrier oil before using.

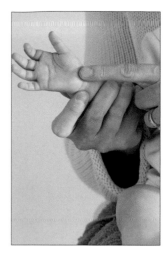

Do a patch test before using an aromatherapy oil in a massage oil: add a drop of the diluted oil to your child's wrist and wait 24 hours to see if any reaction occurs.

them is to dilute them well in a carrier (such as olive oil, sunflower oil or full-fat milk) and then apply the aromatic oil to the skin or mix into the bathwater. Another very gentle way of using them is in a vaporizer.

Always use pure essential oils, preferably those that are made from organically grown plants. Do a patch test on your child before using aromatherapy oils in massage oil: if there is a reaction, it is best to avoid using that essential oil on your child for now. If the skin is fine, that particular oil is safe to use but you will have to test any others in the same way.

Lavender and chamomile are very gentle essential oils and can be used on children over three months.

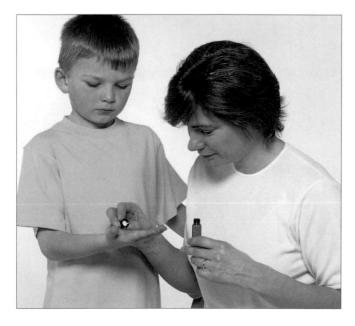

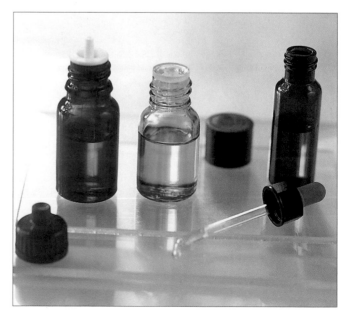

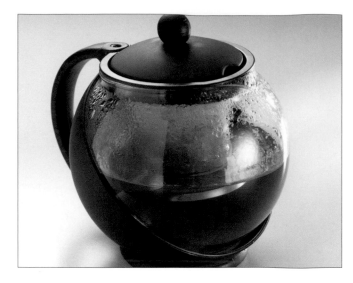

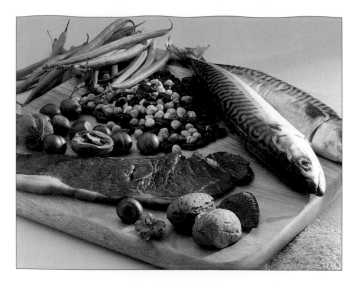

Herbal infusions are a gentle way of giving herbs to a child. The tea should be weak enough to be palatable, you can sweeten it with honey for an older child.

A nutritional therapist can help you to ensure that seemingly healthy food in your child's diet is not the root cause of a lingering health problem.

MEDICAL HERBALISM

Herbal medicine is the oldest form of medicine. Many conventional medicines are based on isolated plant ingredients, but herbalists believe that it is better to use whole parts of the plant – roots, leaves, berries, seeds and so on. The idea is that the many active ingredients in plants work together to promote healing in a gentle and holistic way.

Childhood complaints such as skin problems, asthma, coughs and colds can all be helped with herbal medicine. As with homeopathy, a herbalist will take into account your child's personality and behaviour traits as well as the symptoms when prescribing a remedy.

Herbal remedies come in the form of creams, tinctures, syrups and capsules. Some have well-known effects and can be used in home treatment. But many herbal

remedies can be toxic so it is essential that you do not give one to your child unless you know it to be safe. If your child suffers any ill effects when taking a herbal remedy, stop giving it immediately and contact your herbalist and your doctor.

ACUPUNCTURE OR ACUPRESSURE

These Chinese therapies are based on the idea that well-being depends on the free flow of life energy (chi) through the body. In acupuncture, fine needles are inserted – usually painlessly – into specific points on the body in order to release blockages or quicken a sluggish flow. However, the points can also be stimulated by finger pressure (acupressure), and most acupuncturists would treat children in this way rather than with needles.

The principles that underlie acupuncture are very different to those that inform western medicine, but scientific research has shown it to be highly effective in easing pain and reducing the symptoms of common problems such as constipation, sleeplessness or anxiety. Many doctors are now happy to refer patients to acupuncturists for treatment.

NUTRITIONAL THERAPY

Good diet is fundamental to a healthy life, but particular foods can sometimes be the underlying cause of many childhood complaints: for example, a series of ear infections may be linked to an intolerance of dairy foods. A nutritional therapist will help you to ascertain whether your child is intolerant of particular foods, or deficient in certain nutrients.

You will usually be asked to complete a diet and lifestyle questionnaire before the first appointment. A nutritional therapist may carry out tests, and will come up with an eating plan tailored to your child's particular

MAKING A HERBAL INFUSION

To make a herbal tea for a child over one year, put ¼ tsp dried leaves or ⅓ tsp fresh leaves in a cup or small teapot. Pour over 200ml/⅓ pint boiling water and cover. Leave to steep for 10 minutes, then strain. Give a small cupful (about 50ml/2fl oz) to your child.

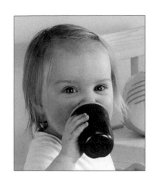

Store the rest in a sterilized screwtop jar in the refrigerator and use within 24 hours. Give no more than three cups a day.

If you want to add the infusion to your child's bath, make ten times the quantity.

NATUROPATHY

Naturopaths use a wide range of natural treatments, including nutritional therapy, herbal remedies and water treatments (hydrotherapy). Some naturopaths may also be trained in homeopathy or osteopathy.

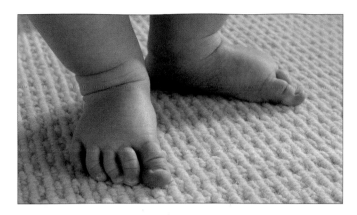

Children can respond well to reflexology, a gentle treatment that uses the soles of the feet to access energy lines within the body. It is a therapy that can benefit even very young children.

needs. He or she may recommend eliminating certain foods for a while and then re-introducing them to check for intolerances. You will usually have to return for several appointments during this process. You may also be given natural supplements such as grapefruit-seed extract for your child to take.

CRANIAL OSTEOPATHY

Cranial osteopaths believe that many physical health problems can result from tiny misalignments in the bones of the skull. They use very gentle touch to manipulate the bones and surrounding tissues into their correct place. Some also practise cranial-sacral therapy, which involves working on the spine and sacrum as well as the head.

SEEING A PRACTITIONER

A complementary health practitioner should take a full medical history of your baby or child from you before starting any treatment. He or she will also ask about various aspects of your child's daily lifestyle and habits: such as bowel movements, sleep patterns, diet, likes and dislikes, and general behaviour. The treatment should always be gentle, and you should be able to stay with your child throughout. After the treatment, symptoms may occasionally get worse for a day or two before they start to improve. Call the therapist or your doctor if anything unusual occurs that worries you. Most therapists recommend several follow-up treatments.

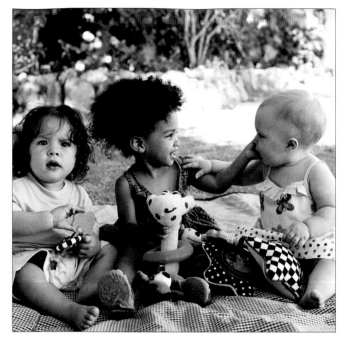

One of the benefits of osteopathy, reflexology, and other natural therapies, is that the therapist can come to your home, which means your child will feel happy, relaxed and secure in their own environment.

Cranial osteopathy and cranial-sacral therapy are particularly good for babies, especially those who have had difficult births. A baby's head is naturally compressed as it travels down the birth canal, and then gradually regains its normal shape over the next few days. Cranial osteopaths say that sometimes this process leaves slight distortions in the skull that cause tension in the body and may be a root cause of sleeplessness, colic, wind and other digestive problems in babies. They believe that it can also be the cause of problems such as recurrent ear infections, frequent blocked-up noses and headaches in young children.

Cranial osteopathy and cranial-sacral therapy are widely used on babies and young children. These treatments are very safe in the hands of a qualified practitioner. However, always go to a qualified osteopath for treatment, not all cranial-sacral therapists have had the rigorous training that osteopaths have.

REFLEXOLOGY

Like acupuncture, reflexology works on energy points. It is based on the idea that the body is divided into ten energy zones, which run from head to feet, and that all the parts of the body can be influenced by working on the feet. Practitioners use a variety of gentle massage techniques to stimulate energy points here, and the effect is generally very soothing.

Reflexology can be good for colic, bowel problems and digestive complaints, skin problems, breathing disorders, sleeplessness and hyperactivity.

Natural first aid

All children have tumbles and minor accidents, and you are bound to have to deal with grazed knees, burns and cuts. Natural remedies help speed healing and can also soothe an unhappy child. But don't hesitate to get medical attention if your child has had a bad fall or if you cannot easily treat the injury yourself.

A NATURAL FIRST-AID BOX

These are some of the most useful natural remedies to have to hand.

Aloe vera gel. A herbal remedy for burns and rashes. Aloe vera has natural antiseptic, antibiotic and anti-inflammatory properties. You can also use the fresh sap of an aloe vera leaf.

Arnica. This homeopathic remedy

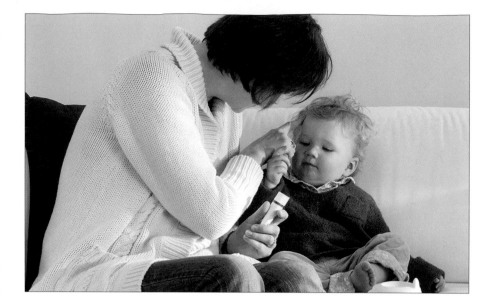

STANDARD FIRST-AID ITEMS

You can buy a first-aid kit from pharmacists, but it is easy to make your own. Get a rigid, closable box and fill it with the following basic items: scissors, safety pins, tweezers, cotton wool, bandages, absorbent dressings, gauze dressings and assorted plasters.

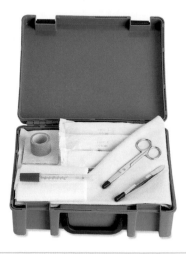

comes in cream and tablet form, and it is worth getting both. The cream is good for bruises; the tablets are also helpful for bruises as well as sprains, shock after an injury, and nosebleeds.

Calendula cream. A natural antifungal and antiseptic cream that fights infection. Calendula is good for minor skin complaints such as burns, blisters and insect bites and stings.

Chamomilla. A homeopathic remedy for teething pain and sleeplessness. Diluted chamomile tea can also be useful, both to sip and for compresses.

Distilled witch hazel. A widely available liquid herbal remedy that is good for bites, stings, bruises and sprains.

Lavender oil. A multipurpose essential oil that has antibacterial and anti-inflammatory qualities; it is good for sleeplessness, minor skin problems and headaches.

Rescue Remedy. This gentle blend of flower essences is great for calming upset children after an accident. Put four drops in water and give to your child to sip.

Most children enjoy having a "magic" cream smoothed over their hurts. Arnica will help to speed healing from bruising.

Roman chamomile oil. A soothing essential oil that helps with sleeplessness, muscle strain and skin problems.

Tea tree oil. An antibacterial and antifungal essential oil that helps to prevent infection.

Honey has been used for centuries as a natural antiseptic, it also has anti-inflammatory qualities, and is a natural antihistamine.

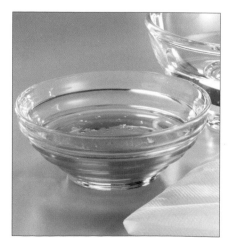

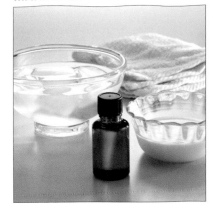

1 Fill a bowl with very cold water and add a handful of ice cubes.
2 Add a few drops of lavender oil diluted in 15ml/1 tbsp full-fat milk.
3 Dip a clean facecloth into the scented water.
4 Squeeze out excess water and apply to the bruised area. Dip the cloth frequently to keep it cold. Apply for a maximum of 10 minutes in total. Reapply every few hours as necessary.

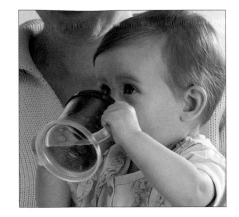

A few drops of Rescue Remedy added to a cup of water can help soothe minor shocks and upsets.

CUTS AND GRAZES

Most cuts are minor wounds that heal quickly but you should always clean the damaged skin to prevent infection. Grazes often occur when the child has slid along the ground after a fall, so they may contain bits of dirt or grit, which will all need to be removed.

What to do. Fill a small bowl with warm water, add a couple of drops of tea tree oil and use to bathe the wound, or simply wash under running water. Press a folded pad of gauze or similar over the area to stop bleeding (don't use cotton wool (cotton balls) as the fibres may stick). Smooth a little Calendula cream over the cleaned area before covering with a plaster. You can also apply honey: ideally use manuka honey, which has a marked antibacterial and anti-inflammatory action.

When to seek help. Seek medical attention if the cut is very deep, there are objects embedded in it that you cannot easily remove, it doesn't stop bleeding when a dressing is applied or if it covers a large area.

BRUISES

When the blood vessels under the skin are damaged, blood seeps out into the surrounding tissues, causing bruising. Some children bruise more easily than others. Including more fruits and vegetables in the diet can help, since these foods are known to contain vitamin C and bioflavonoids, which help to strengthen the walls of blood vessels.

What to do. Apply a cold lavender compress to the skin for a few minutes to reduce swelling. A packet of frozen peas wrapped in a towel will also work well. Don't hold a compress against your child's skin for longer than 10 minutes. To encourage healing, smooth Arnica cream on the bruise three times a day. You can also give an Arnica tablet immediately after the injury to help with the shock, and every two hours during daytime for the next 48 hours.

When to seek help. See a doctor if you suspect a broken bone, or if the pain is worse 24 hours later. Frequent bruising is occasionally due to a problem with blood clotting: see your doctor if your child bruises very easily and unusually.

NOSEBLEEDS

A nosebleed happens when the delicate blood vessels that line the nose are damaged by a blow, frequent nose-blowing or picking, or inflammation caused by a cold. If your child has nosebleeds often, try giving more fruits and vegetables to increase his or her intake of vitamin C and bioflavonoids.

What to do. Get your child to lean forwards (not backwards), and gently pinch the fleshy part just under the bridge of the nose for 10–15 minutes. Release, repeat if bleeding continues. Arnica tablets can be given after a nosebleed, or daily for frequent bleeds. Rescue Remedy helps soothe any shock.

When to seek help. Take your child to hospital if a nosebleed occurs after a blow to the head, or if the bleeding doesn't stop within half an hour. See a doctor if your child has frequent nosebleeds.

A pack of frozen peas wrapped in muslin makes a makeshift icepack.

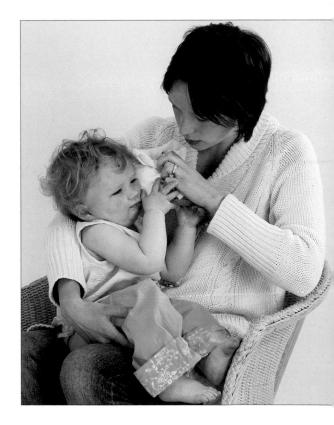

CHOKING

A sudden fit of coughing may mean your child is choking on a piece of food or other small item. The natural instinct to give someone who is choking a slap on the back is a good one, but encourage a child to cough first – this is often enough to remove an obstruction. Check the mouth and remove the obstruction if you can see it: don't feel for it with your fingers – you may damage the throat or push the obstruction in further.

If you do need to slap the child on the back, get him to bend over (or bend him over your knee) and slap between the shoulderblades. If a baby is choking, hold him face-down along your forearm so that the head is facing downwards and use two fingers to tap sharply between the shoulder blades.

All parents worry about choking and it is worth learning how to do chest compressions and life-saving procedures in the very unlikely event that back slaps don't clear the obstruction. You can do a simple first-aid course specifically for babies and children; this usually involves practising the techniques on a life-sized model. Courses are run by voluntary organizations such as St John Ambulance (Red Cross) and are aimed at parents and carers. Often there are child care facilities.

SPRAINS AND STRAINS

A sprain is an injury to the ligaments of a joint, while a strain is an injury to a muscle. It's quite difficult to tell the difference between a strain or sprain and a fracture, especially in young children, whose bones may bend rather than break. If in doubt, seek medical advice.

What to do. Get your child to sit or lie down. Apply a cold lavender or chamomile compress or ice pack for up to 10 minutes. Place a thick wad of cotton wool or other soft pad against the injury and bandage firmly, or put on an elastic bandage to compress. Then elevate the

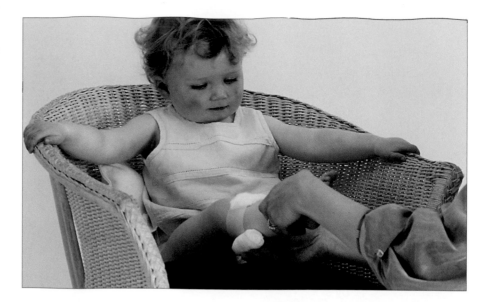

injured part to reduce swelling. Give Arnica for shock and to encourage healing; Rhus tox is another good homeopathic remedy for sprains and strains. Apply Arnica cream or comfrey ointment over the area (only if the skin is unbroken). Rescue Remedy will help soothe any upset.

Caution. Be sure that you do not bandage so tightly that you cut off the circulation. To check, press on an uninjured area of skin below the bandaged area. If it takes more than three seconds for colour to return, your bandage is probably too tight.

When to seek help. Get medical advice if you suspect a fracture or if the pain doesn't subside at all after the treatment.

WASP AND BEE STINGS

These stings can be very painful.
What to do. If you can see a sting in

Arnica cream and tablets help to speed healing for a strain or sprain.

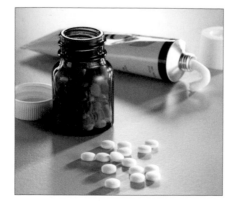

If you need to bandage a sprain, use a thick wad of gauze or cotton wool to cushion the wound first.

your child's skin, remove it carefully. Put a little iced water in a bowl and add a few drops of lavender or tea tree oil diluted in 15ml/1 tbsp full-fat milk. Dip cotton wool in the water and apply to the area every 10 minutes or so until the pain subsides. Other easily available natural remedies for bee stings include witch hazel, bicarbonate of soda or crushed garlic; wasp stings can be helped by applying witch hazel, cider vinegar or lemon juice. The homeopathic remedy Apis can be given to help with the after-effects of a sting.

When to seek help. If your child is allergic to wasp or bee stings, he or she may go into anaphylactic shock, needing urgent medical attention.

INSECT BITES

Gnat, ant or mosquito bites can be very itchy.
What to do. Witch hazel is a good treatment for insect bites. Rescue Remedy can be applied to the bite. Mosquito bites can be soothed with cider vinegar or lemon juice.
Prevention. Before dusk, when mosquitoes are most active, cover up your child in clothes of closely woven, lightly coloured fabric. You can get eucalyptus-based repellents

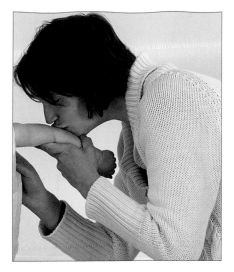

Remove a bee sting by scraping it off with a credit card or by pressing your thumb into the neighbouring skin and pushing it sideways. Don't try to pull it out with tweezers: this can squeeze any poison left in the sting into your child's skin. Suck out any poison before treating.

suitable for children from health food stores. Burning citronella oil in a vaporizer or using citronella candles is also helpful.

BURNS

Minor (first-degree) burns affect only the top layer of skin, which reddens but does not blister or swell. They can be treated at home.

What to do. Place the burned area under cold, running water for 10 minutes. Apply aloe vera gel, Calendula cream, or lavender oil

Acidic lemon juice or cider vinegar can take the sting out of a mosquito bite.

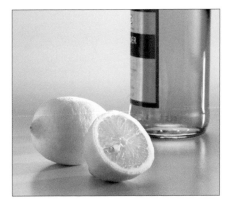

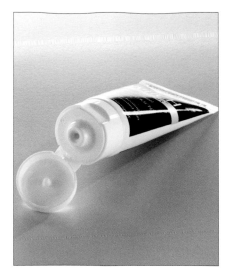

You can get witchhazel in the traditional tincture form or in handy tubes of gel.

diluted in full-fat milk to ease pain and speed healing. Give Rescue Remedy or Arnica for the shock.

When to seek help. If the burn is larger than the child's palm or if the pain gets worse after treatment, seek immediate medical advice. If the skin is moist, swollen or blistered, the burn may have reached underlying areas of skin (second-degree burn); if the child feels no pain after a burn but the area is red, white, yellow or darkened, the nerves may be damaged (third-degree burn). Seek urgent medical advice.

SUNBURN

It's important to protect your child's delicate skin from the sun. If it gets too much sunlight, the skin will be red, hot and sore.

What to do. Bathe the skin in cool water to which you have added a couple of drops of lavender oil diluted in full-fat milk. Add a few drops of lavender oil to aloe vera gel and smooth over the affected area. The homeopathic remedy Sol is good for mild sunburn.

When to seek help. Seek immediate medical advice if the skin has blistered, or if your child develops a high temperature (39°C/102°F or above).

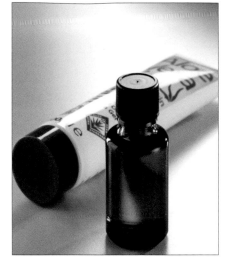

Aloe vera gel and lavender essential oil are two natural remedies for minor burns.

SUNSTROKE

A sunburned child may also develop heatstroke, with a raised temperature, headache, nausea, dizziness and general aches.

What to do. Cool your child down by sponging with tepid water. Give plenty of cool drinks to sip: water, diluted fruit juice or a rehydration drink (available from pharmacists). The homeopathic remedies Sol or Belladonna may be given.

When to seek help. Get immediate medical help if your child's temperature is very high (39°C/102°F).

FOREIGN OBJECTS IN THE EYE

Children can easily rub grit or other irritants into their eyes.

What to do. If you can see a piece of grit in your child's eye, get the child to put his or her head on one side with the affected side uppermost. Holding the eyelids open with your fingers, very slowly pour tepid water into the upper corner of the eye so that water covers the whole eye. If the grit doesn't move, try lifting it off with the corner of a damp handkerchief.

When to seek help. Seek immediate medical attention if something is stuck to the surface of the eye or embedded in it.

When your child is sick

As your child gets older, it becomes easier to assess what is wrong: now he or she can point to a sore throat, or tell you exactly where it hurts or how they feel. You will still have to rely on the outward signs of illness, too, however. If your child is unusually irritable, not interested in eating or suddenly drinking more than usual, something may be wrong.

You will probably have a good sense of how poorly your child is. Don't hesitate to contact your doctor if you think the child may be seriously ill or if you are not sure what is wrong. If you think the illness may be infectious, tell the reception staff who can arrange for you to sit away from other patients.

CARING FOR A POORLY CHILD

Rest is the best way of managing most illness. If your child doesn't want to stay in bed, then let him or her sit with you: read stories, do jigsaws or simply let the child nap on the sofa. Put light, comfortable clothing on your child: pyjamas and a light cardigan or dressing gown. If the child is in bed, change the sheets regularly. Open the window from time to time to air the room. Disinfect the room using a natural spray (see box).

Be prepared for your child to revert to babyish behaviour traits: a young child who is just potty-trained, for example, may revert to nappies. Be patient if he or she is fractious and irritable.

SYMPTOM SORTER

Symptoms with or without fever	Could be
Runny nose, cough or sneezing	Cold
All the above plus aches and pains	Flu
Sore throat and pain on swallowing	Throat infection
Runny or blocked nose, pain in ear or (in young child) crying and pulling on ear	Ear infection
Cough, phlegm	Bronchitis
Cough, phlegm and /or rapid or difficult breathing	Bronchiolitis
Itchy red spots that blister	Chickenpox
Frequent urination and pain or burning when passing water	Infection in urinary tract
Diarrhoea and/or vomiting	Food poisoning or gastroenteritis

If your child has a fever, take steps to reduce it. Give lots of fluids, preferably water with a little added fresh lemon juice. Failing this, try diluted fruit juice even if you don't usually give it: juice is a good way to get vitamins into your child and encourage him or her to drink.

Children who are poorly often don't want to eat. This won't harm your child, and it's best not to encourage eating: his or her body may need to put all its energy into

WHEN TO SEEK HELP

Contact a doctor if your child:
- has an unexplained rash
- has a high or persistent fever
- is breathing very fast or noisily
- is unusually sleepy and cannot be roused
- is making you feel concerned.

Go to hospital or call an ambulance if your child:
- cannot breathe properly
- has a fit or is unconscious
- has severe leg pain, cold hands or feet with a high body temperature, very pale skin or blue-tinged skin around the lips (early signs of bacterial meningitis)
- has a headache, stiff neck, aversion to bright light or a purplish-red rash that does not disappear when pressed with a glass (later signs of bacterial meningitis)

AIR FRESHENER

For a natural room spray to refresh the air in your child's room, use 5 drops each of lavender, thyme linalol and eucalyptus smithi essential oils to 150ml/$\frac{1}{4}$ pint water. Pour into a plant spray bottle, shake well, and spray into the air.

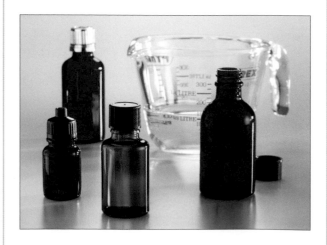

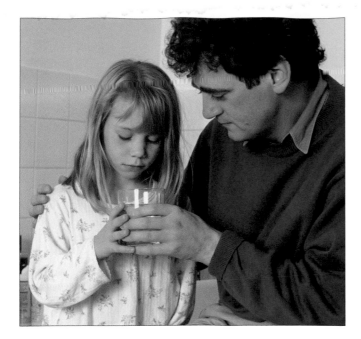

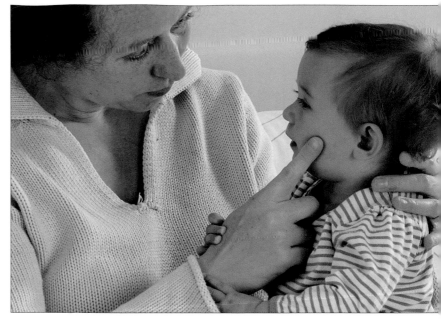

Being sick and having diarrhoea dehydrates the body, so make sure your child drinks enough water after vomiting. Encourage them to take small sips of cooled, boiled water and repeat at intervals.

Trust your own instincts: if something tells you that your child is seriously ill, act on your intuition. You know your child better than anyone else, so you may pick up on clues that may not be obvious to other people.

fighting off an infection. Once your child starts to feel better, the appetite may return. Give foods that are easy to eat and gentle on the stomach: a thick, smooth home-made vegetable or chicken soup, mashed potato, natural yoghurt with mashed-up banana, or a smoothie made with fruit juice, yoghurt and honey.

A HOSPITAL STAY

A stay in hospital is bound to be disorientating and intimidating for a young child. Prepare your child as much as you can by talking about what will happen. Sharing a book about a child who has to go to hospital could help. If possible, go on a visit to the ward where your child will be staying – see if he or she can meet some of the nurses and other staff who work there and see some of the fun things – such as the television above each bed. Be as matter-of-fact as you can: it is important that your child

doesn't pick up on your anxiety. But do acknowledge any feelings of fear or worry your child may have.

Take familiar items with you: your child's favourite toy or comforter, pyjamas, bowl and spoon, as well as the essentials. Take snacks, water, a book and comfortable clothing for yourself as well. Stay with your child in hospital: even if you have to sleep in an armchair, it will make your child feel much better if you are there. If you cannot be there all the time, ask another trusted relative or friend that the child knows well to fill in for you. Make sure that you are present when your child is examined by a doctor. Even if your child seems to cope well with being in hospital, don't be surprised if he or she displays some signs of disturbance once you get home. It is common for children to be clingy or naughty, even aggressive, after an unsettling experience. Be patient and this will pass.

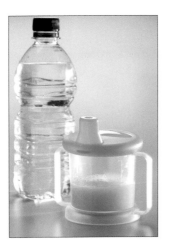

Left: Diluted juice is a good way of boosting a poorly child's energy levels. Use freshly squeezed juice if you can; it has more nutrients.

Right: During illness or convalescence, tempt a poor appetite with food that is easy to eat – a banana and yoghurt smoothie is ideal.

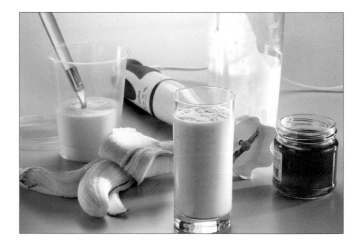

Common problems: colds, coughs and breathing disorders

Children get more coughs and colds than adults. Most children catch between six and eight colds a year until they build up immunity. And as the airways of a child are much smaller than those of adults, they are more vulnerable to infection.

COLDS

It is viruses that cause colds, so antibiotics do not help. A cold usually lasts a week or two, but can go on for longer in young children. Symptoms include a blocked-up or runny nose, sticky eyes, sore throat, a tickly cough (especially at night) and slight fever.

What to do. You can't hasten a cold's progress, but you can make your child more comfortable. Keep him or her warm, but open windows regularly to get fresh air circulating. Take your child out (well wrapped up) on short trips. Increase the humidity in the child's room to help with breathing: put a damp towel on the radiator, place a bowl of water near the radiator or other heat source or use a vaporizer.

Give lots of fluids. Children over a year old can have hot honey and lemon, which is soothing for the throat and a good source of vitamin C. Weak elderflower tea acts as a decongestant. Dilute fruit juices can also be a good way of encouraging a child to drink. Unsweetened blackcurrant diluted with warm water is good if your child has a cold: it is packed with vitamin C.

- If your child is eating, cut out dairy products (which are mucus-forming) while symptoms remain, but give alternative sources of calcium such as tofu, ground nuts and seeds, and leafy green vegetables. Babies will still need their usual milk.
- Get older children to blow their nose regularly, to stop mucus dripping down the back of the throat.
- Consider giving a homeopathic remedy to soothe symptoms. The following are common cold remedies: Aconite, given in the first 24 hours; Allium cepa, when there is lots of watery discharge from the nose and eyes; Pulsatilla, when there is thick, greenish mucus.

When to seek help. Seek medical advice if you spot other unusual signs, such as wheezing or earache, if the symptoms are very severe or if your child gets more poorly after a few days.

COUGHS

Coughing is how the body removes irritants or mucus from the breathing apparatus, so it is best to avoid over-the-counter medications that are designed to suppress this natural mechanism. If your child suddenly starts coughing violently, consider whether he or she may have inhaled a foreign object. Take steps to remove it from the airway (see first aid for choking).

What to do. If your child is coughing, the suggestions given for colds above are helpful, together with the following:

- Humidify all rooms by placing a bowl of water under the radiator or heat source.
- Avoid taking your child outdoors if the weather is cold and damp.
- For babies over three months, put a drop of essential oil of

For colds, give drinks of diluted blackcurrant, orange or lemon juice sweetened with a little honey.

There are many homeopathic remedies for different types of cough and cold symptoms.

Eucalyptus oil is a good natural decongestant, but you need only a drop on a tissue.

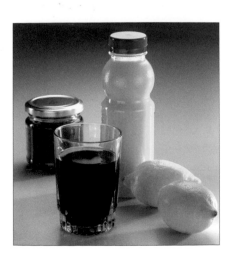

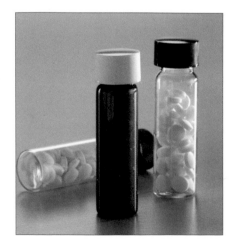

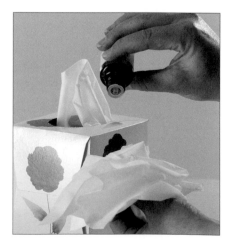

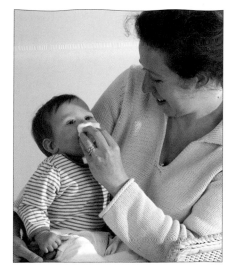

Use soft cotton wool (cotton balls) rather than tissues to wipe a child's nose to stop it getting sore.

eucalyptus smithi (not eucalyptus globulus, which is stronger) on a handkerchief and leave it in your child's room, out of reach.

- For children over one year, give diluted warm blackcurrant juice to soothe a sore throat, or thyme tea remedy (see box). If children are eating, include mild spices such as cinnamon or ginger in their food to help loosen mucus. Pineapple is also good because it contains bromeline, which is a natural anti-inflammatory.

- Consider giving one of the many homeopathic remedies used to relieve symptoms. A homeopath will help you pinpoint the right one for your child. Common remedies include: Aconite, for a dry cough that comes on at night; Bryonia, for a dry, painful cough (worse on inhalation) that follows a cold; Ipepac, for a cough that is accompanied by vomiting up phlegm; Phosphorus, for a dry, tickly cough that is worse at night; Pulsatilla, for a cough that produces yellow or green phlegm.

When to seek help. Coughing can be a minor ailment or a symptom of some much more serious illnesses such as bronchiolitis and bronchitis. Always see a doctor if a cough occurs in a young baby, or if it is severe, prolonged or accompanied by wheezing, noisy breathing or fast breathing.

CROUP

A barking cough and noisy breathing on inhalation are the key signs of croup, which is most common among children aged between six months and three years.

What to do. There are two ways to improve the breathing: take your child into a steamy room (run the hot shower and taps in the bathroom to create steam) or wrap the child up well and go outside into the cold air. Different approaches work for different children, so do which works best for your child.

THYME TEA REMEDY

This traditional remedy can help to ease a dry cough and loosen mucus. If possible, use New Zealand manuka honey, which has particular therapeutic properties.

Add a small handful of finely chopped thyme leaves to a cup of boiling water, steep until cool, then strain. Add honey to sweeten, then pour into a sterilized jar. Give 1 tsp three or four times a day. Keep in the refrigerator for up to 3 days.

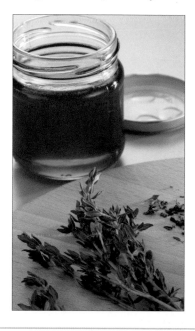

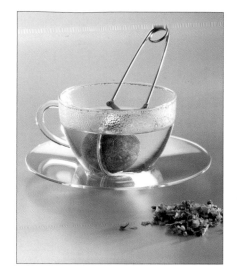

For flu, try giving your child weak lime flower tea, which helps to treat fever and reduce nasal catarrh.

BRONCHIOLITIS

This viral infection is most common in babies under twelve months, and affects the smallest airways in the lungs (the bronchioles). It starts as a cold and fever and develops into coughing, fast breathing (more than 50 breaths a minute) and wheezing.

What to do. See your doctor quickly: sometimes hospital treatment is needed.

BRONCHITIS

This infection of the large airways (bronchi) is common in toddlers and children. The symptoms are similar to those of bronchiolitis. Deficiencies in vitamin C and zinc can be an underlying cause for recurrent lung problems such as bronchitis.

What to do. Medical advice should be sought. Giving a multivitamin multimineral supplement in addition may help.

FLU

The symptoms of flu include a high temperature, aches and pains, cold symptoms, vomiting and/or diarrhoea and general malaise.

What to do. See your doctor for a diagnosis. Lime flower and elderflower tea – or a combination of both – are good for flu. They should be drunk warm, well diluted.

Common problems: asthma and eczema

Asthma and eczema are now very common in young children. Both are the result of oversensitivity of the immune system, which cause it to react to substances that have no effect on other people. They often occur together, and affected children are also more likely to suffer from food allergies.

Nobody quite knows why asthma and eczema have become so prevalent, but it may be because improved living standards have reduced the amount of germs children come into contact with, with the result that their immune systems are less robust. The increase in pollution, both outdoors and indoors, is also a likely factor. One Australian study found that exposure to the volatile organic chemicals (VOCs) found in paint and other

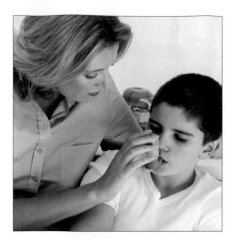

Asthma medicine is given via an inhaler and can quickly reduce symptoms of an attack. Children using inhalers need supervising by a responsible adult.

products increased the risk of childhood asthma. Exclusive breastfeeding in the first months of life can reduce the likelihood of both asthma and eczema developing.

ASTHMA

Growing numbers of children suffer from the recurrent attacks of breathlessness and wheezing that characterize asthma. In asthmatic children, the small airways in the lungs are hypersensitive: they narrow when they come into contact with, say, small amounts of smoke or pollutants. Asthma usually gets better as the child gets older. A child who is diagnosed with asthma will be given inhalers to prevent attacks and relieve symptoms. Natural therapies can help to support conventional medical treatment.

What to do. Try to identify possible triggers for your child's asthma and take steps to avoid them. Your doctor can arrange tests to check for allergy to substances such as dust mites. Improve the air quality in your home and keep it free of dust (but

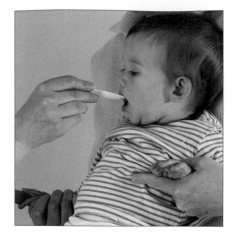

Fish oils have been shown to ease symptoms of both asthma and eczema. In one study, three out of four children given fish oil found that their symptoms improved.

vacuum when your child is out of the way). Choose a synthetic pillow and duvet with allergen-proof covers for your child's bed, and wash the bedding often in hot water. Limit toys in the cot to one or two, and wash them each week at 60°C/140°F or put in a plastic bag in the freezer overnight to kill dust mites.

Make sure that your child has a healthy diet including lots of fresh fruits and vegetables: this has been shown to be good for lung function. Choose organic produce wherever possible to reduce your child's exposure to pesticides. Do not put salt in your child's food, and avoid processed foods that contain added salt and additives such as tartrazine, which may exacerbate asthma. Consider consulting a nutritional therapist to help you uncover any possible food intolerances, and give a multivitamin, multimineral supplement: low levels of vitamin C, vitamin B6, vitamin B12, magnesium and zinc can exacerbate the symptoms. Homeopathy may help. Arsenicum, Ipecac, Nat sulph and

CHECKLIST OF ASTHMA TRIGGERS
- Dust mites
- Pollen
- Pet dander (animal hair and skin scales)
- Certain foods, especially eggs, dairy products, chocolate, wheat, citrus fruits and corn
- Mould spores
- Colds and other respiratory infections
- Cigarette smoke or exhaust fumes
- Fumes from air fresheners, household cleaners, perfumes, dry-cleaning solvents, paints, glues and pesticides
- Cold air
- Exercise
- Stress and anxiety.

Pulsatilla are all prescribed to relieve mild asthma attacks, but you should see a homeopath for a specific remedy for your child. Herbal medicine has several remedies for asthma. A medical herbalist can advise you on the best herbs to use (alongside conventional treatment). Acupuncture may be helpful for some asthma sufferers, and yoga or breathing exercises may help.

ECZEMA

There are different types of eczema: those that usually affect children are seborrhoeic eczema (cradle cap) and the itchy atopic eczema, which one child in five develops. Atopic eczema can affect any part of the body, but is most common on the face, armpits, elbows, hands and knees. During an acute attack, the skin reddens, becomes extremely itchy and can blister and weep. It may be thick, dry and flaky at other times.

What to do. See your doctor, as it's essential to manage your child's eczema to prevent infection. Eczema reduces the skin's ability to act as a barrier, and bacteria are more likely to stick to dry, flaky skin.

Avoid irritating the skin. For example, choose clothing or bedding made from cotton, launder

Keep your child's fingernails short to stop him or her scratching areas of skin affected by eczema and causing infection.

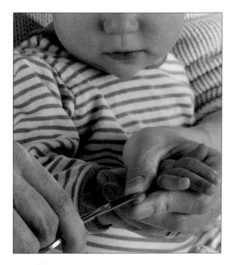

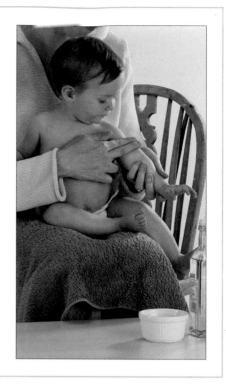

OILS FOR ECZEMA
Aromatherapy oils may help with mild eczema symptoms. Try this simple recipe. You can also make a cool compress using the same oils to soothe itching.

2 drops chamomile essential oil
2 drops lavender essential oil
45ml/3 tbsp hypoallergenic lotion

Mix together all the ingredients and then apply to the affected skin in a thin layer. Be sure to do a patch test 24 hours before you first use the lotion.
You can also make a cool compress using the same oils diluted in a simple carrier oil such as olive oil to soothe itching.

with non-biological washing powders and use an extra rinse cycle on your washing machine. Avoid soap and bath products. Keep your child as cool as possible, as heat and sweating exacerbate eczema. Cut his or her fingernails short to help prevent scratching (put cotton mittens on babies and young children at night).

Keep your child's skin clean and moisturized. Give lukewarm (not hot) daily baths to remove dry skin scales and cleanse the skin. Use an emollient such as a handful of oatmeal tied in a muslin square (you can add a drop of lavender or chamomile essential oil). Different creams work for different children. Hemp seed oil cream is one good natural alternative to try, as is olive oil. Apply a thin layer and let it soak in rather than rubbing it in (which can increase itching).

Increase oils in your child's diet. Add a spoonful of hemp seed oil to your child's food each day and give oily fish or a supplement. Give lots of water to keep your child well hydrated. Consider food sensitivity as an underlying factor, and see a qualified nutritional therapist to help

you pinpoint any problem foods. Milk, wheat, nuts, citrus fruits, fish and eggs are the most likely culprits, and sugar can exacerbate eczema. As with asthma, a multivitamin, multimineral supplement may be helpful, and a child-friendly probiotic will help to improve the balance of good bacteria in the gut, which can also be beneficial.

A probiotic drink that is suitable for children may help with eczema.

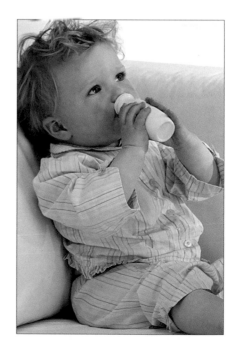

Common problems: digestive disorders

Children have sensitive digestive systems that react quickly to get rid of unwanted substances: they are much more prone to diarrhoea and vomiting than adults. These unpleasant symptoms are basically the body's way of cleansing itself, so medications to stop them are generally unhelpful. Your main aim should be to reduce discomfort and prevent dehydration.

Tummy ache is unusual in very young children, so it is best to report it to a doctor to rule out the possibility of appendicitis. In older

Most children become distressed after vomiting. Give your child a glass of cool water to sip: add a few drops of Rescue Remedy to calm and reassure.

children, it can have a physical or emotional cause: gastroenteritis, overeating or anxiety can all be responsible. Sometimes it can be triggered by other infections, such as tonsillitis. Call a doctor if your child is in severe pain, there is blood in his or her stools or if tummy ache and fever occur together.

DIARRHOEA
Your child may get a short bout of diarrhoea (frequent, loose, unpleasant-smelling stools) after having a lot of fruit or fruit juice, after eating a food he or she is intolerant to, when teething or with a cold. A course of antibiotics can also be a trigger. Diarrhoea can be a sign of food poisoning or gastroenteritis, especially if accompanied by

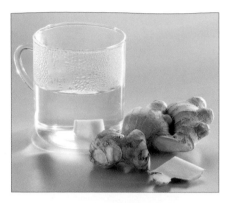

Fresh ginger is a natural remedy for nausea. All you need do is steep a piece of the fresh root in a cup of hot water for a few minutes.

vomiting. In most cases, it lasts 24 hours or less and clears up by itself. **What to do.** Give frequent drinks for sipping. Let a nursing baby breastfeed on demand and give a bottle-fed baby extra drinks of cooled, boiled water. Plain water should be sufficient in mild cases, but you can also give a rehydration drink (available from pharmacists) if necessary. Antispasmodic herbal teas, such as chamomile or fennel, can ease abdominal pains. Diluted unsweetened blackcurrant juice helps to fight infection in the gut.

For a soothing tummy massage, add one drop chamomile essential oil to 15ml/1 tbsp olive or sunflower oil. Gently massage the tummy, with clockwise circular strokes.

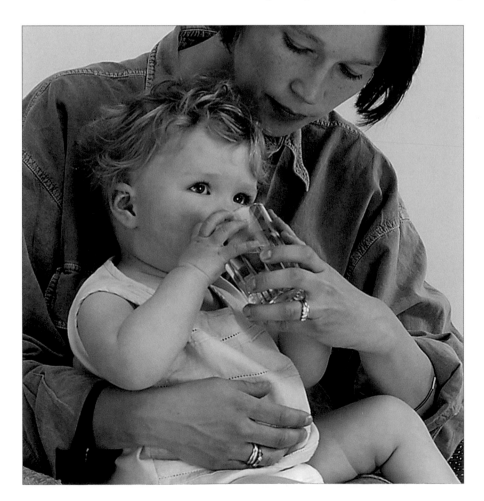

DEHYDRATION
Seek immediate help if your child shows signs of dehydration: dry mouth, sunken eyes, loose skin and dry nappies. The soft spot on the top of a baby's head (the fontanelle) may become depressed.

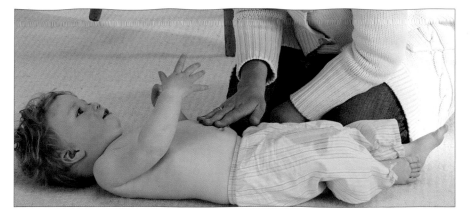

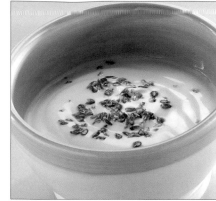

A gentle tummy massage, following the path of the intestines, can help to get the bowels moving.

Fibre-rich ground flaxseed can help with constipation. Add a little to natural yoghurt or a smoothie.

Consider giving a suitable probiotic to help balance the bacteria in the gut. This can help reduce the duration of a bout of diarrhoea. If the diarrhoea occurred after you introduced a new food into your child's diet, make a note of it. If the symptoms re-occur the next time you give the food, then your child is almost certainly sensitive to it and it is best avoided.

When to seek help. Contact a doctor if a baby has diarrhoea for more than a few hours or if it lasts longer than 24 hours in an older child. Also, seek medical help if the diarrhoea is very severe, if there is blood in the stools, if your child seems dehydrated or has persistent stomach ache or if you think he or she has taken something toxic.

VOMITING

Like diarrhoea, vomiting can have many causes. If your child is doing both, the most likely cause is gastroenteritis or food poisoning. Vomiting on its own can be the result of the child having eaten too much (or a baby having taken too much milk) or can be part of a feverish illness. A baby with a cold may be sick, to expel phlegm from the body.

What to do. Treat as for diarrhoea (but avoid giving a tummy massage). Encourage your child to sip rather than to gulp liquid to help it stay down. Ginger is particularly good for

nausea and vomiting: you can make a simple ginger tea by steeping a block of peeled, bruised garlic in a cup of hot water.

When to seek help. Contact your doctor if a baby vomits repeatedly or violently, or if vomiting and diarrhoea occur together. Seek medical advice for an older child if vomiting is very frequent, lasts longer than 24 hours, or if there is blood in the vomit.

CONSTIPATION

If your child suddenly goes for longer than normal between bowel movements, and then produces hard, dry, pebble-like stools, he or she is constipated.

What to do. Increase the vegetables and fruits in your child's diet (but cut out bananas): broccoli, leafy green vegetables and dried apricots are particularly helpful. Give older children whole grains: porridge oats and rye bread are better than wholewheat bread, which can irritate the lining of the gut. Most important

If your child is hungry after vomiting or diarrhoea, plain boiled rice is very gentle on the stomach.

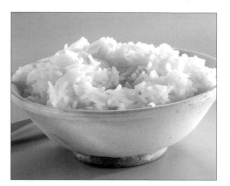

of all, make sure your child is well hydrated: give extra cups of water and remind the child to drink them.

Consider sprinkling a little ground flaxseed (available from health food stores) on your child's cereal, or put 5ml/1 tsp flaxseed oil into your child's food or in a fruit smoothie. Flaxseeds are rich in fibre and are a natural lubricant. Give live yoghurt if the balance of the intestinal flora has been upset by a bout of gastroenteritis or a course of antibiotics. Or consider giving a child-friendly probiotic supplement.

Massage can soothe cramping and encourage the bowels to move: stroke your hand over the abdomen, making an arch shape in a clockwise direction so that you are following the line of the intestines. For children over one year, you can use a massage oil of orange essential oil diluted in a carrier oil. Reflexology treatment can be helpful: one Scottish study found that regular treatment helped to relieve chronic constipation in children.

If constipation is a recurring problem, consider whether food sensitivity could be a root cause. An Italian study found that sensitivity to cow's milk caused chronic constipation in some children.

When to seek help. Seek medical advice if your child does not have a bowel movement for several days, or if the problem is recurrent.

Common problems: skin rashes and ear infections

Rashes are a feature of many childhood infections, both non-serious and serious. It's quite hard to distinguish between different rashes, so it is best to check them out with your doctor.

CHICKENPOX

The first symptoms of chickenpox are usually tiredness, fever and loss of appetite. Within a day or two, small, flat red spots appear, usually on the back, stomach and chest. They can spread to the face and head in a day or two. The red spots join up and blister, becoming intensely itchy. They scab over within 24 hours, as more spots appear.

Chickenpox is infectious from two days before the spots appear until scabs have formed on all the spots. It takes 10–21 days for the symptoms to appear after infection. One attack usually confers lifelong immunity. Chickenpox can be very dangerous for unborn children if the mother is not immune, so if your child has been in contact with a pregnant woman, let her know, so that she can contact her doctor.

Chickenpox spots blister and then scab. They are itchy, but discourage your child from scratching in case of infection and scarring.

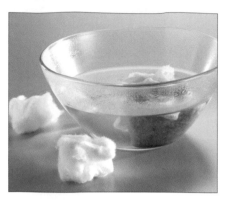

Make an elderflower infusion, dip cotton wool in the bowl and dab on the spots for relief from itching.

What to do. Encourage your child to rest as much as possible and take steps to manage any fever. Use calendula cream or calomine lotion on the spots to relieve itching, or dab them with elderflower tea or a solution of 5ml/1 tsp distilled witch hazel in a cup of warm water. Give lots of fruits and vegetables to boost your child's immune system, and add raw garlic to food if your child will eat it. Consider giving the following homeopathic remedies:

- Aconite, for the initial symptoms of tiredness and fever
- Belladonna, for the early stages if temperature is high and the child is flushed and very thirsty
- Rhus tox, for itching and any restlessness.

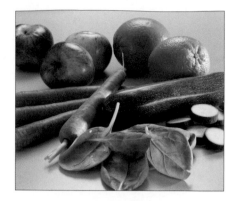

Encourage your child to eat lots of healthy fruits and vegetables to promote healing.

Protect your child's skin from direct sunlight for a couple of weeks after the scabs fall off, to avoid any danger of scarring.

When to seek help. See your doctor if a baby is affected, if the attack is severe, if the spots become inflamed or if you are pregnant and are not sure that you are immune.

HEAT RASH

Young children have immature sweat glands, which are easily blocked. Heat rash usually appears as small red bumps, sometimes with a blister in the centre, that appear on areas exposed to sunlight or areas that sweat a lot.

What to do. Cool your child down: remove clothing, sponge down or give the child a tepid bath. Good topical treatments include aloe vera gel, distilled witch hazel, Calendula cream or a lavender or chamomile compress. The homeopathic remedy Sol can also be helpful.

IMPETIGO

This infectious skin condition usually starts off around the mouth or nose. It takes the form of red blisters, which soon burst and form a golden crust on reddened, weeping skin.

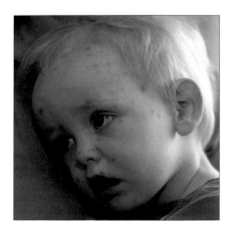

> **RELIEVING ITCHING CHICKENPOX SPOTS**
> A lukewarm oatmeal bath can be soothing. Place a handful of oatmeal in a muslin square or the foot of a nylon stocking, add 2 drops each of chamomile and lavender essential oils, tie up and place in the water. Give several baths a day.

GLUE EAR

This is a condition in which thick, sticky fluid accumulates in the middle ear, leading to hearing problems. It can be linked to repeated ear or throat infections, which block the Eustachian tube. If it is persistent, the conventional treatment is the insertion of a plastic grommet to allow fluid to drain. But the procedure involves a general anaesthetic and has itself been linked to hearing problems. Repeated ear infections are often a cause, so take steps to avoid them (see above). Many complementary health practitioners believe that glue ear is linked to food sensitivity, particularly an intolerance of dairy foods, or to passive smoking.

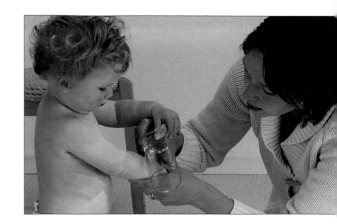

What to do. Bathing the skin with warm salt water can help to reduce itching; tea tree oil added neat to water can also help with itching and can limit the infection. Give garlic perles every two hours for a day or two, then reduce to three times a day, to help resolve the infection. The homeopathic remedies Ant crud or Arsenicum can be useful.

Be scrupulous about hygiene: do not share face towels or pillows and keep your child away from other children while infectious.

EAR INFECTIONS

Children are prone to ear infections, particularly after a cold or throat infection. The Eustachian tube, the drainage canal that links the nose, ear and throat, is very narrow. If it becomes blocked, fluid accumulates and viruses and bacteria multiply. The main symptoms are pain, hearing loss and fever. A small child

Warmth can soothe the pain of an earache; use a covered hot water bottle or a lavender compress.

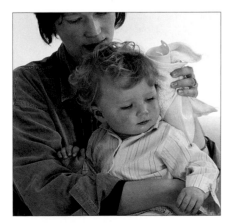

may tug on the ear, but most simply cry and seem unwell.

Seek medical advice straight away if you suspect your child has an ear infection. It needs prompt treatment – usually antibiotics – to prevent the infection spreading. Take steps to prevent recurrence, so your child does not have to take repeated courses of antibiotics.

What you can do. Warm the affected ear by holding a warm lavender compress or a covered hot-water bottle against it. Dilute lavender essential oil in olive or sunflower oil and smooth into the skin around the ear and neck.

For children over one year, give plenty of warm drinks such as honey and lemon and fresh blackcurrant juice; you can give a herbal tea combining chamomile (antiseptic and relaxing), elderflower or lemon balm (to reduce mucus) and lime flowers (to bring down fever) three times a day. Garlic can help relieve infection: add fresh garlic to your child's food if possible, or give garlic perles. If your child has taken antibiotics, give live yoghurt every day for a month to help rebalance the bacteria in the gut.

Raise the head of the cot or bed to help fluid drain from the Eustachian tube. Avoid washing your child's hair or going swimming while symptoms persist. Consider giving a homeopathic remedy, such as:

- Aconite, at the onset of symptoms, especially if the child has a blocked nose, fever and is thirsty
- Belladonna, for earache that is

To test for a meningitis rash, press a clear glass against it. If the spots do not disappear seek immediate medical aid.

worse at night and better when the child sits upright
- Chamomilia, for earache that accompanies teething, is causing extreme pain and irritability
- Pulsatilla, for earache with a cold that is worse at night.

If your child gets repeated ear infections, keep his or her ears, throat and neck warm at all times: wrap the child up well in cold weather. Give the remedies mentioned above at the first signs of a cold, to try to head off infections, but seek advice from a homeopath for a remedy specifically tailored to your child. Consider food sensitivity as a possible cause. Dairy products are the most common culprits, but wheat, eggs and chocolate could also be triggers in some children.

Make sure your child is eating a healthy, balanced diet, with plenty of fresh fruits and vegetables, zinc-rich foods such as meat and poultry, and lots of garlic. Do not give sugar, which depresses the immune system. Warm drinks of honey and lemon or diluted fresh blackcurrant juice support the immune system and encourage mucus to clear. Consider giving a multivitamin, multimineral supplement.

When to seek help. See a doctor if you suspect an ear infection, or if blood or clear liquid is discharged from the ear.

Food allergy and intolerance

Though often confused, food allergy and food intolerance are two different things. In food allergy, the immune system mistakenly identifies the food as a foreign invader. This can cause an extreme and sometimes life-threatening reaction. Food allergy may affect up to 8 per cent of children, but most grow out of it: just 2 per cent of adults are affected. Children with a food allergy are more likely to suffer from other allergy-related problems such as eczema or asthma, which also tend to diminish with age.

Food intolerances are harder to pin down. Symptoms vary widely, even in the same individual. They are usually milder and can occur hours or days after the food is eaten. Some may be delayed reactions by the immune system, others are caused by the body's inability to digest the food properly. For these reasons, many doctors are sceptical even about the existence of many food intolerances, while many nutritional therapists believe them to be a factor in a wide range of common childhood ailments.

WARNING

Children with severe allergies can go into anaphylactic shock, in which their blood pressure drops and they become unconscious. Anaphylaxis can be fatal unless the victim is treated with a shot of adrenaline (epinephrine): call an ambulance immediately. Parents and teachers of children with a severe allergy need to carry an adrenaline shot with them so it can be administered at any time.

COMMON FOOD ALLERGENS

Any food can trigger a reaction, but about 90 per cent of food allergies are caused by one of the following eight foods:

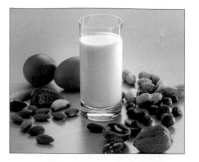

Cow's milk; eggs; peanuts; wheat; soya; tree nuts (such as walnuts, brazil nuts, hazelnuts, almonds and pecans);

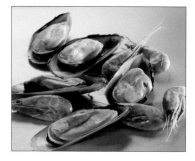

Fish and shellfish.

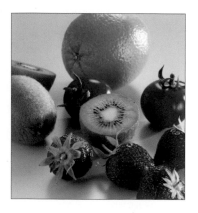

Other common allergenic foods include strawberries, kiwi fruit, tomatoes, oranges, and chocolate.

SYMPTOMS

Common symptoms of food allergy include:
- swelling of the lips and throat
- skin rash, eczema or itching
- swelling of the eyelids
- vomiting or diarrhoea
- wheezing or breathing difficulties.

If a child is intolerant – as opposed to allergic – to a food, the symptoms are usually more general, though some are similar to those of an allergic reaction. They include:
- fatigue
- vomiting and diarrhoea
- bloating and wind
- eczema or skin rashes (especially around the mouth)
- wheezing
- muscular aches and pains
- frequent colds or ear infections
- temper tantrums or behaviour problems
- sleeplessness
- cravings (perhaps for the very food the child is intolerant of).

WHAT TO DO

If you suspect that your child may be allergic to a food, the first step is to visit your doctor to arrange for a test. Tests usually take the form of a blood test or a prick test (in which the skin is scratched and a tiny amount of the allergen introduced to see if a reaction occurs). If your child tests positive for an allergy, the only option is to cut the food out of the diet and replace it with healthy alternatives. If there is any doubt, an elimination diet can determine the suspect food. Cutting a food out of the diet is not as easy as it sounds. Someone with an allergy to soya, for example, will also need to avoid foods labelled tempeh, tamori, textured vegetable protein, and so

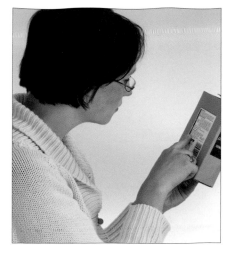

If your child has a food allergy, you will get used to reading the lists of ingredients on food labels: many problem foods crop up in a surprising variety of forms and names. You can find information on food labelling on food allergy websites.

on. A dietician can tell you what you need to look for on food labels.

It is more difficult to test for food intolerances than allergies. As a starting point, try keeping a food diary for two weeks, listing everything your child eats and any symptoms. This can sometimes help you to get a better idea of whether

Sweets are full of colourings, preservatives, sugars and artificial sweeteners, all of which can cause behavioural reactions, and certainly have no nutritional value.

your child does indeed have a food intolerance.

If you think this is the case, see your doctor and asked to be referred to an allergy specialist or a dietician. An allergy specialist can help you to check for intolerance by removing the suspect foods from your child's diet for five to ten days, and then re-introducing them. The short period of abstinence should be scrupulously observed in order to be sure that all traces of the food have passed through the digestive system. This has the effect of making any reaction when the food is re-introduced stronger and more immediate, making diagnosis easier.

Although the process sounds simple, it is best to have professional advice when you undertake it: it is very easy to make the mistake of assuming a child has a food intolerance when this is not the case, which could lead you to restrict his or her diet unnecessarily. A specialist will also help ensure that your child is getting essential nutrients while following an exclusion diet.

Where an intolerance is diagnosed, eliminating the problem food is the usual remedy, as with allergies. However, in the case of intolerance, when a food is excluded from the diet, the body tends to build up tolerance to it. This means that the child may be able to eat it again in small quantities not too frequently.

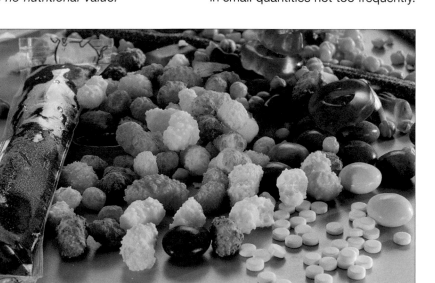

ELIMINATING FOODS
Don't be tempted to exclude important foods such as milk from your child's diet without professional advice. It can be difficult to provide alternative sources of, say calcium. Children can become malnourished while following a severely restricted diet.

If your child does have a food sensitivity, make sure he or she has a good balanced diet, and takes regular meals and snacks to keep blood-sugar levels steady. Consider giving a multivitamin, multimineral supplement and a suitable probiotic drink to encourage good digestion. It's important to get your child to chew food properly (this makes it easier to digest).

You can help to build your child's tolerance to a problem food such as wheat by eliminating it from the diet for a couple of months. After this, the child may have no trouble eating occasional pieces of bread.

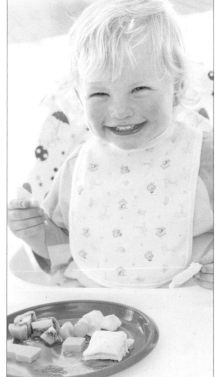

A healthy home

We are all exposed to toxic chemicals every day: they are in the air we breathe, our food and drink and the toiletries and household products we use. Because our homes are enclosed spaces, toxin levels can build up and the air can actually be more polluted than it is outdoors. Ordinary household dust can contain a mixture of solvents, hormone-disrupting chemicals, heavy metals, solvents, pesticides and flame retardants. Children spend a lot of their time indoors and they are more likely to be affected by pollution than adults. So it is important to ensure that your home is a healthy environment for your child to grow up in.

Here are some basic steps for a healthy home.
• Ban smoking at home.
• Open your windows regularly.
• Keep pets out of sleeping areas. If your child is allergic to your pet, you may have to keep it out of all living areas or find it a new home.
• Wipe your feet when you come in, and leave your shoes by the door to avoid bringing dirt, heavy metals and toxic chemicals indoors.
• Choose furniture made from untreated natural materials.
• Wash curtains, other soft furnishings and bedclothes regularly.

Keeping your home dust-free will help to protect your child from inhaling pollutants. But use natural products rather than spray polishes and carpet cleaners.

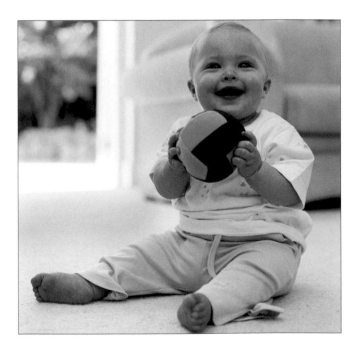

NATURAL CLEANING PRODUCTS

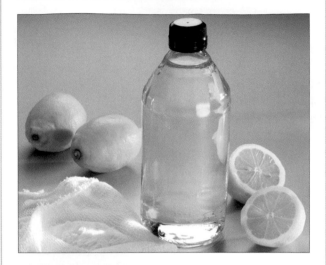

You can use ordinary ingredients to tackle many cleaning jobs around the home.

Bicarbonate of soda (baking soda). Sprinkle this on a damp sponge and use to clean surfaces. For stubborn stains, mix it with a little water and leave for 20 minutes before wiping off. Add 30ml/2 tbsp bicarbonate of soda to a cup of vinegar and add to the toilet bowl. Leave for at least 15 minutes, then clean with a brush. To clean a drain, add half a cup of bicarbonate then half a cup of vinegar. Leave for 15 minutes, then pour down a kettle of boiling water.

White vinegar. This is great for cleaning windows. Add half a cup of vinegar to 1 litre/2 pints warm water and apply with a soft cloth, then buff with crumpled newspaper. Vinegar can also be used for descaling appliances: add equal parts of vinegar and water to a kettle and leave overnight. Throw out the vinegar, boil the kettle and discard the water before using again.

Lemon juice. Lemon is an excellent natural brightening agent and cleanser. Add half a cup of lemon juice to a bucket of water and soak white or coloured clothes overnight before washing as usual.

• Keep your home as dust-free as possible. Consider buying a vacuum cleaner with a high-efficiency particulate air (HEPA) filter. Keep children out of the way while you dust and vacuum.
• Dry clothes outside or in a properly ventilated space. Avoid putting them around the house (on radiators and so on); the moisture will be released into the air and may cause the growth of mould spores in your walls.

DECORATING

If you are planning a nursery for your baby or revamping a child's bedroom, seek out non-toxic decorating products and furnishings. Babies and children spend a lot of time on or near the floor, so choose a natural covering such as wood or cork rather than laminate or vinyl, which may contain harmful chemicals. Hard flooring is the best option because carpet traps dust, which can lead to a build-up of airborne toxins and dust mites. But if you want to use carpet for warmth, choose wool, sisal or coir with a natural backing, and vacuum regularly.

Regular paints contain volatile organic compounds (VOCs), which give off noxious vapours after being applied. Choose water-based low-VOC paints, keep the room well ventilated during and after decorating and don't let your child sleep in the room for a few days after painting it. Better still, use organic paints made from natural materials such as linseed, casein and mineral pigments. These take longer to dry and can be harder to use, but they are safe for allergy- and asthma-sufferers.

If you are picking furniture for a child's room, avoid items made from MDF, laminated wood or chipboard, which contain formaldehyde. Choose furniture made from untreated hardwood from sustainable sources instead. Use natural materials for your child's bedding. For example, get a mattress made from organic latex, wool and cotton, and sheets of unbleached organic cotton.

CUT THE CHEMICALS

Reducing the amount of chemicals you use in the home will lower the risk of your child coming into contact with something harmful.

- If your kitchen cupboard is a jumble of different products, go through it and get rid of any products you don't use. General cleaners may leave a residue on your surfaces, which your child may then touch: so avoid those labelled 'irritant' and choose gentle eco-friendly products or natural cleaning alternatives instead.

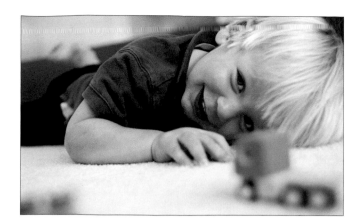

Young children inevitably spend a lot of time on the floor, so it is worth investing in natural coverings that are free from unnecessary chemicals.

- In the same way, go through your bathroom cupboards and throw out any products that you do not need. Avoid wearing perfume, hairspray and a plethora of other products to reduce the amount of chemicals your child breathes in. He or she will prefer your natural smell in any case. Put only natural substances on your baby or toddler – he or she can do without bubble baths, wipes, talc and harsh soaps.
- Get rid of garden pesticides, weed killers and so on. Many common garden products – including creosote – have now been banned, so it is best to dispose of any products you have had for several years. Consider gardening organically to help protect your child from hazardous chemicals. For example, use saucers of beer sunk into the soil to trap slugs rather than poisonous pellets (which a young child could eat).

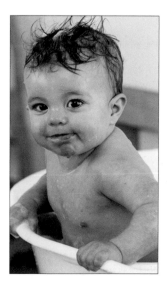

Left: Avoid using unnecessary toiletries. Many bubble baths contain detergent, which irritates the skin, while the ingredients for baby wipes may include propylene glycol – a chemical that is also present in anti-freeze.

Right: Make sure your child spends some time outside every day, whatever the weather.

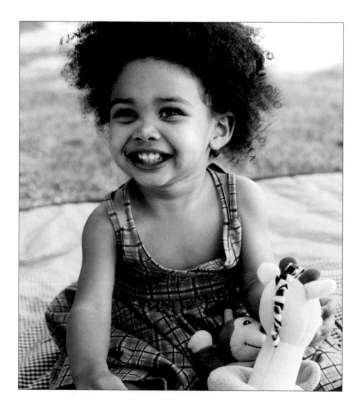

Safety in the home

Young children are naturally curious and have little sense of danger, so it is up to you to make their environment safe. To make your home child-friendly, you need to develop an eye for potential disaster. The best way to do this is to crawl around so that you see each room from a child's perspective. Notice what dangles down, what can be pulled or poked, opened or climbed, and then take steps to make it safe. Be prepared to refine your childproofing at the major stages of your child's development – crawling, walking and so on.

Young children need constant adult supervision: they shouldn't be left in a room alone even for a few minutes. Take extra care when you are under pressure, entertaining guests or trying to get ready to go out: accidents are more likely to happen when you are distracted. It's a good idea to get your child used to a playpen from an early age, so that you have somewhere to put him or her when you need to concentrate on something else.

KEEPING ACTIVE CHILDREN SAFE

- Fit stairgates at the top and bottom of stairs once your child is ready to crawl.
- Check your banisters are safe: you need vertical spindles no more than 10cm/4in apart.
- Put locks on any windows that your child could open.
- Make sure that the locks on external doors are set higher than your child can reach. If not, fit a high bolt.
- Put plug covers on all unused electrical sockets. Turn off the switch at the socket when you are not using it.
- Cover any child-level glass with safety film.
- Put corner covers on any tables.
- Attach freestanding bookshelves to the wall.
- Constantly check floors and other areas for small items that your child could choke on: coins, marbles, pen tops, buttons, rubber tyres from toy cars, small squidgy balls and burst or uninflated balloons are all potential hazards to your child.

IN THE BEDROOM

Children's bedrooms are usually safer than other parts of the home, because they are decorated and furnished with the child in mind. Keep these basic things in mind:

- Make sure your child's cot is a safe place. The bars should be no more than 7cm/2¾ in apart, and the mattress should fit snugly. Don't give a child under one year a duvet or pillows.
- Position the bed away from windows and radiators.
- Don't put anything under the window (such as low

FIRE!

Smoke inhalation, burns and scalds are all common injuries in childhood. Contact your local fire service for individual advice on protecting your home from fire (fire officers may be willing to fit smoke alarms free of charge).

- Don't overload sockets.
- Don't use an extension lead that isn't powerful enough for the appliance; large appliances should not be plugged into extension leads. Put extension leads away after use.
- Don't leave candles or aromatherapy vaporizers that use a naked flame burning: it's safest not to use them at all. Get in the habit of putting matches and lighters well out of reach.
- Do put smoke alarms on every floor; install a carbon monoxide alarm too.
- Do cover all open fires with a fixed fireguard. Use radiator covers too.
- Do switch off appliances at the socket when they are not in use.

Babies and young children love to rummage through handbags. Be on the safe side and don't ever keep sharp items such as nail clippers or scissors in yours, and make sure any medications you use are in child-safety containers.

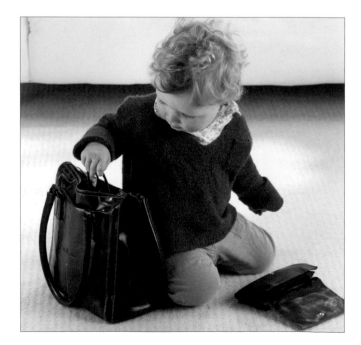

cupboards, bookshelves or toy boxes) that your child could use as a step. Don't forget to fit window locks in your child's room.

- Use a radiator cover to protect your child from burns. Alternatively, turn the thermostat down and cover the radiator with a large towel.

IN THE KITCHEN

The kitchen is full of items that are potential hazards for inquisitive children. You need to get into the habit of tidying up after yourself and closing cupboard doors and drawers once you have got what you need. If you can, keep your child out of the kitchen when you are cooking: you may be able to use a stair gate to fence off the cooking area or fit in a playpen to keep your child safe.

Store plastic bags and clingfilm out of reach: young children instinctively want to wear a bag like a hat. Keep knives somewhere safe. Fit locks to low-level cupboards and drawers. Store dishwasher tablets (which are particularly noxious) and other cleaning products in a locked cupboard, and make sure that your child knows this is the "nasty cupboard". If a child does swallow something toxic, get medical advice urgently. If you need to go to hospital, take the packaging with you.

When you are cooking, turn saucepan handles to the back of the hob, and use the rear burners when possible. Hob guards can make cooking and lifting pans awkward, so are not advisable. Give up deep-fat frying, which is very dangerous, or invest in an electric fryer. Have a small fire extinguisher and a fire blanket to hand.

The best time to iron is when your child is in bed. If you iron at other times, keep your child away (in a playpen or behind a safety gate) and put the iron out of reach when you have finished. Put it away when it is cool.

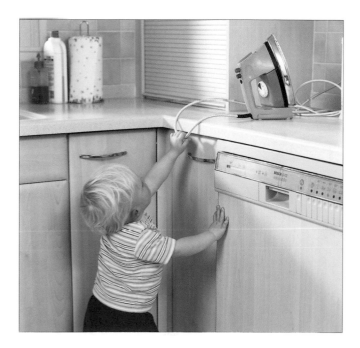

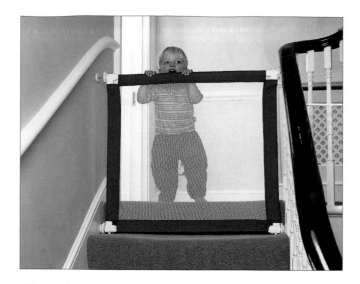

Fit a stairgate at the top and bottom of stairs until your child can safely navigate them independently. Let children practise going up and coming down from time to time: teach your child to come down bottom first.

Put the kitchen bin somewhere your child cannot access. Clean up spills quickly, to avoid slipping, and watch for toys, particularly wheeled ones, left in the kitchen. Ban tablecloths for now, and push chairs in under the table so that your child doesn't use them as a step.

IN THE BATHROOM

Supervise young children at all times when they are in the bath and don't leave a filled bath unattended: a child can drown in even shallow water and your toddler may be better at climbing than you think. If you need to do something, get your child out of the bath and take him or her with you.

Keep the toilet seat cover down. A toilet seat lock is useful. Keep mouthwashes, cleaners, razors and all types of medicines in a locked cabinet. Get rid of glass thermometers that contain mercury; take them to a pharmacist for safe disposal. Consider turning the hot water temperature down to less than 55°C/130°F.

SAFETY WITH TOYS
- Don't let your child play with a toy intended for an older child; age ranges are recommended for safety reasons.
- Don't give toys with long strings to a baby: they are a strangling hazard. Musical cot toys with strings should be removed before the child can get on hands and knees.
- Remove all packaging and labels before giving a toy to your child.
- Check second-hand toys carefully. Old toys may have been made to less stringent safety standards.
- Get rid of broken toys that cannot be repaired.

Useful addresses

UK
Allergy UK
3 White Oak Square
London Road
Swanley, Kent, BR8 7AG
Tel: 01322 619898
www.allergyuk.org

Asthma UK
Providence House
Providence Place
London N1 0NT
Tel: 08457 01 02 03
www.asthma.org.uk

Child Accident Prevention Trust
22-26 Farringdon Lane
London EC1R 3AJ
Tel: 020 7608 3828
www.capt.org.uk

Eneuresis Resource and Information Centre
Tel 0845 370 8008
www.eric.org.uk
Advice on bedwetting and soiling

Gingerbread
7 Sovereign Close
Sovereign Court
London E1W 3HW
Tel: 0800 018 4318
www.gingerbread.org.uk
Local support groups for single-parent families

Institute for Complementary Medicine
Tel: 020 7231 5855
www.icmedicine.co.uk

National Association of Toy and Leisure Libraries
68 Churchway
London NW1 1LT
Tel 020 7387 9592

National Childminding Association
8 Masons Hill
Bromley, Kent BR2 9EY
Tel: 0800 169 4486
www.ncma.org.uk
Advice on finding a childminder

National Eczema Society
Hill House
Highgate Hill, London N19 5NA
Tel: 0870 241 3604
www.eczema.org

St John Ambulance
27 St Johns Lane
London EC1M 4BU
Tel: 020 7324 4000

www.sja.org.uk
Information on first aid courses

Single Parents Action Network
Millpond, Baptist Street
Easton, Bristol BS5 0YJ
Tel: 0117 9514231
www.spanuk.org.uk

Other useful websites
www.mothering.com
www.raisingkids.co.uk

USA
American Holistic Medical Association
PO Box 2016
Edmonds, WA 98020
Tel: 425.967.0737
www.holisticmedicine.org

American Red Cross
2025 E Street, NW
Washington DC 20006
Tel: 202 303 4498
www.redcross.org

Food Allergy Initiative
1414 Avenue of the Americas,
Suite 1804
New York, NY 10019
Tel: 212-207-1974
www.foodallergyinitiative.org

National Safekids Campaign
1301 Pennsylvania Avenue NW
Suite 1000,
Washington DC 20004
Tel: 0202 662 0600
www.safekids.org

CANADA
Food Allergy and Anaphylaxis Campaign
11781 Lee Jackson Hwy, Suite 160
Fairfax,
VA 22033-3309
Tel: 800 929 4040
www.foodallergy.org

Safe Kids Canada
180 Dundas Street W
Toronto,
Ontario K1G 5L5
Tel: 416 813 7288
www.safekidscanada.com

St John Ambulance Canada
1900 City Park Drive, Suite 400
Ottawa,
Ontario, K1J1A3
Tel: 613 236 7461
www.sja.ca

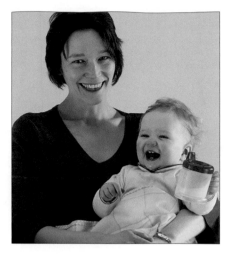

AUSTRALIA
Anaphylaxis Australia
21 Robinson Close
Hornsby Heights, NSW 2077
Tel: 1300 728 000
www.allergyfacts.org.au

Australian Complementary Health Association
247 Flinders Lane
Melbourne, Victoria 3000
Tel: 03 9650 5237
www.diversity.org.au

Kidsafe Australia
50 Bramston Terrace
Herston, Queensland 4029
Tel: 07 3854 1829
www.kidsafe.com.au

St John Ambulance
PO Box 3895
Manuka, ACT 2603
Tel: 1300 360 455
www.stjohn.org.au

NEW ZEALAND
Allergy New Zealand
PO Box 56 117
Dominion Road, Auckland
Tel: 09 303 2024
www.allergy.org.nz

St John Ambulance
Level 11, St John House
114 The Terrace, PO Box 10 043
Wellington
Tel: 04 472 3600
www.stjohn.org.nz

Safekids New Zealand
PO Box 26488
Epsom, Auckland
Tel: 09 630 9955
www.safekids.org.nz

Index

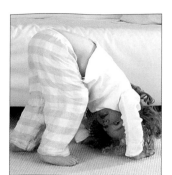

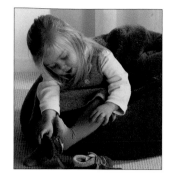

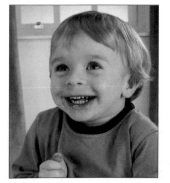

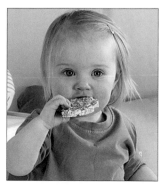

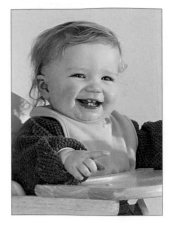

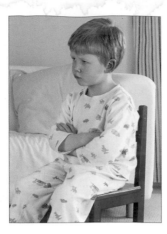
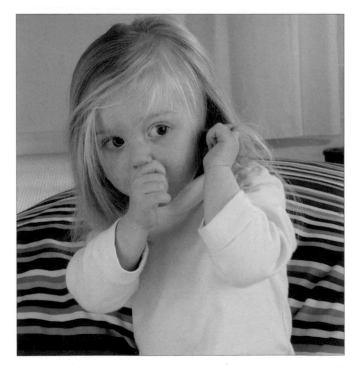